DATE DUE

JAN 3 1 1995	
FEB 1 5 1995	
NOV 2 0 1995	
FEB 1 9 1996	
APR 2 3 1997	
AUG 2 6 1997	
MAR 1 0 1998	
APRIL 09/98	
APR 2 9 1998	
OCT - 9 1998	
NOV 2 4 1999	
FEB 2 4 2001	
DEC 3 2001	
APR - 3 2002	

BRODART.   Cat. No. 23-221

Orthopaedic Surgery

The material contained in this book is endorsed by AORN as a useful component in the ongoing education process of perioperative nurses.

MOSBY'S PERIOPERATIVE NURSING SERIES

Orthopaedic Surgery

Brenda Gregory, RN, BSN, CNOR

Clinical Supervisor, Operating Room
Memorial Hospital Southeast
Houston, Texas

*with **570** illustrations*

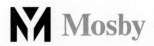 **Mosby**

St. Louis Baltimore Boston Chicago London Madrid Philadelphia Sydney Toronto

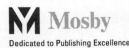

Mosby
Dedicated to Publishing Excellence

Editor: Michael S. Ledbetter
Developmental Editor: Teri Merchant
Project Manager: Gayle May Morris
Production Editors: Judith Bange and Donna L. Walls
Design Manager: Susan Lane
Book Design: Jeanne Wolfgeher
Manufacturing Supervisor: Betty Richmond

Printed in the United States of America
Composition by Graphic World, Inc.
Printing/binding by Von Hoffmann Press, Inc.
Color separation by Color Associates, Inc.

Mosby–Year Book, Inc.
11830 Westline Industrial Drive
St. Louis, Missouri 63146

Library of Congress Cataloging in Publication Data
Gregory, Brenda.
    Orthopaedic surgery/Brenda Gregory.
      p.   cm.—(Mosby's Perioperative nursing series)
    Includes bibliographical references and index.
    ISBN 0-8016-6552-3
    1. Orthopedic nursing.   2. Orthopedic surgery.   I. Title.
  II. Series.
    [DNLM: 1. Orthopedic Nursing—methods.   2. Orthopedics—methods.
  WY 157.6 G822o 1994]
  RD753.G74   1994
  617.3—dc20
  DNLM/DLC
  for Library of Congress   93-31530
                                       CIP

94 95 96 97 98 / 9 8 7 6 5 4 3 2 1

To my father

Always remembered, always loved

A true inspiration

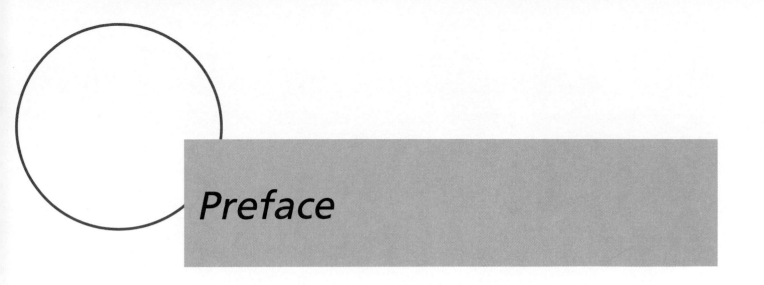

Preface

Perioperative nursing is a unique and challenging career demanding advanced knowledge in the area of speciality practice. The perioperative nurse and other health care providers must be knowledgeable and skilled in basic competencies, as well as surgical procedures and techniques.

Orthopaedic Surgery is a comprehensive reference written with consultation from specialists who serve the orthopaedic patient population. It is designed to provide information on basic surgical interventions and relevant techniques used in orthopaedic surgical nursing. This foundational information will be highly useful to nurses caring for the patient in the preoperative, intraoperative, and postoperative phases. It is also valuable for operating room or radiology technicians, physical therapists, students, and representatives from the health care industry.

Orthopaedic Surgery is divided into two major sections. The first section contains basic principles and technology unique to caring for orthopaedic patients. A summary of the musculoskeletal anatomy, nursing care, instrumentation, and equipment involved in orthopaedic surgical nursing is presented to enhance implementation of care. The second section covers orthopaedic surgical interventions for more than 50

common problems divided into acquired, traumatic, and congenital disorders. Each procedure identifies key steps that will assist the perioperative nurse in patient teaching, assessing and planning use of supplies and equipment, surgical positioning, procedural implications, and evaluation of care. Hundreds of full-color photographs clearly illustrate the key steps of each procedure. The terminology used throughout the book is generic, and the key steps describe common technique.

This book is intended to provide perioperative nurses and others involved in the care of patients undergoing orthopaedic surgery with the knowledge needed to anticipate and plan a patient's care based on a solid understanding of the procedures. In my roles as a clinician, educator, and manager, I sought information that would help me share knowledge and skills to guide others in their practice and help them develop their role as an expert. It is this desire to share information with peers who want to develop an expertise in this distinctive specialty that has made writing this book worthwhile.

Brenda Gregory

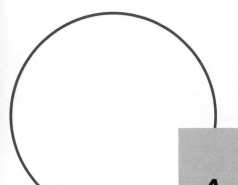

Acknowledgments

The friends and peers who assisted in providing photo opportunities for this textbook are to be commended for their time and effort. Appreciation is extended to Jim Null, Medislide, Inc., for making himself available for unscheduled orthopaedic procedures. I am grateful to Belinda Ischy, surgical technologist, for her capacious love of orthopaedics; and to Emily McDonald, RN, BSN, and the administration of Memorial Hospital Southeast, Houston, Texas, for the opportunity to improve nursing care of patients undergoing orthopaedic surgery. A special thanks to Ernest Beck for use of the many anatomy and physiology illustrations. Appreciation is also given to the following for their generous assistance and various contributions:

Susan S. Ball, RN, BSN
Assistant to J.B. Bennett, MD,
Orthopaedic Surgery,
Houston, Texas

James B. Bennett, MD
Clinical Professor,
Department of Orthopaedic Surgery,
Baylor College of Medicine,
Houston, Texas

W. Grant Braly, MD
Clinical Assistant Professor,
Department of Orthopaedic Surgery,
Baylor College of Medicine,
Houston, Texas

Rebecca P. Chalupa, RN
Staff Nurse,
Scurlock Operating Room,
The Methodist Hospital,
Houston, Texas

Donna K. Dahms, RN, BA, CNOR
Nurse Clinician—Perioperative Education,
Department of Nursing Education,
The Methodist Hospital,
Houston, Texas

Wendell D. Erwin, MD
Clinical Professor,
Department of Orthopaedic Surgery,
Baylor College of Medicine,
Houston, Texas

Gary M. Gartsman, MD
Clinical Associate Professor,
Department of Orthopaedic Surgery,
Baylor College of Medicine,
Houston, Texas

Joseph J. Gugenheim, MD
Clinical Assistant Professor,
Department of Orthopaedic Surgery,
Baylor College of Medicine;
Houston, Texas

Glen C. Landon, MD
Associate Professor of Clinical Practice,
Department of Orthopaedic Surgery,
Baylor College of Medicine,
Houston, Texas

Kenneth B. Mathis, MD
Assistant Professor,
Department of Orthopaedic Surgery,
Baylor College of Medicine;
Staff Physician,
Memorial Hospital Southeast,
Houston, Texas

Melinda Murchison, RN
Operating Room,
Texas Children's Hospital,
Houston, Texas

Keith S. Schauder, MD
Clinical Faculty,
Baylor College of Medicine,
Division of Sports Medicine,
Memorial Hospital Southeast,
Houston, Texas

Susan K. White, RN, BSN, CNOR
Head Nurse,
Scurlock Operating Room,
The Methodist Hospital,
Houston, Texas

Debbie Wooten, RN
Nurse Manager, Orthopaedics,
Texas Children's Hospital,
Houston, Texas

CONSULTANTS

Larry Asplin, RN, RT, CNOR
Northway Surgicenter,
Division of St. Cloud Hospital,
St. Cloud, Minnesota

Joseph P. Dutkowsky, MD
Assistant Professor and Director of Laboratory Research,
University of Tennessee–Campbell Clinic, Department of
Orthopaedic Surgery,
Active Staff—Campbell Clinic,
Memphis, Tennessee

Roxanne Huckstep, RN, AA, BS, CNOR
Orthopaedic Specialist,
Riverside Regional Medical Center,
Newport News, Virginia

Janel P. Nemec, RN, ONC, CNOR
Nurse Clinician,
Orthopaedic Surgery,
Cleveland Clinic Florida,
Fort Lauderdale, Florida

Rhonda Price, RN, BSN
University of Iowa Hospitals and Clinics,
Iowa City, Iowa

Jane S. Witchey, RN, BSN
Charge Nurse, Operating Room,
Santa Barbara Cottage Hospital,
Bath/Pueblo,
Santa Barbara, California

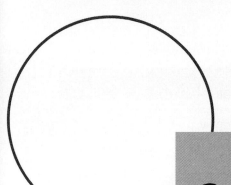

Contents

PART ONE

Foundations of Orthopaedic Surgical Nursing

1 *History of Orthopaedic Surgery* 3

2 *The Orthopaedic Team* 5
Perioperative orthopaedic nurse, 5
Role of the orthopaedic surgeon, 6
Registered nurse first assistant, 6
Anesthesia team, 6
Certified surgical technologist, 6
Other providers, 6

3 *Musculoskeletal Structures* 9
Tissue structure, 9
Skeletal structure, 9
Muscular structure, 25
Bone development and healing, 26

4 *Perioperative Nursing Care* 29
Care for special populations, 29
Communication, 30
Assessment, 31
Diagnosis, 34
Outcome identification, 35
Planning, 35
Implementation, 38
Evaluation, 43

5 *Instrumentation* 47
Care and handling, 47
Basic instruments, 48
Cutting instruments, 48
Bone-holding instruments, 51
Retracting instruments, 53
Nonspecific categories, 53

6 *Equipment and Supplies* 61
Assessment of needs, 61
Types of equipment, 61
Postoperative communication, 69

PART TWO

Surgical Interventions

7 *Acquired Musculoskeletal Disorders* 73
Nursing care, 73
Arthroscopic procedures, 74
Soft tissue procedures, 91
Shoulder repair, 97
Spinal repair, 104
Arthroplasty, 111
Procedures to correct disorders of the foot, 135
Bone graft and stimulation, 140

8 *Traumatic Musculoskeletal Injury* 145
Nursing care, 145
Fracture types and treatment, 151

9 *Congenital Anomalies* 191
Nursing care, 191
Procedures for common anomalies, 193
Spinal instrumentation, 207

PART ONE

Foundations of Orthopaedic Surgical Nursing

1

History of Orthopaedic Surgery

Orthopaedic nursing has evolved as a specialty as a result of the need to refine patient care in a highly specialized area. Orthopaedic surgical procedures are as old an art as medicine itself. Amputations were the first musculoskeletal surgical procedures performed, following the invention of knives and crude saws. The first known written material on surgery of the musculoskeletal system is contained in Egyptian papyri dated about 1600 BC (Breasted, 1922). Two of the Hippocratic books, *On Fractures* and *On Articulations*, from Greece dated between 400 BC and 100 AD. These contain a thorough discussion of the diagnosis and treatment of fractures, including sophisticated methods of traction for the reduction of long-bone fractures.

Galen (131-201 AD), Greek by birth, was one of the first notable clinical investigators. He used his laboratory for extensive studies on blood vessels and was one of the first to understand the function of the musculoskeletal system and to use the terms *kyphosis, lordosis,* and *scoliosis* (Bick, 1968). Paul of Aegina (625-690 AD) described the management of patellar fractures, discussed osteotomy of bones for malunions, recognized the malleability of soft callus, and provided the first description on record of a simple laminectomy (Enneking, 1979).

Minimal progress was made in the field of medicine and surgery from the fifth to the twelfth century. During the twelfth and thirteenth centuries Western civilization emerged, and there was a rebirth of interest in the study of human anatomy. Surgical arts were expanded, cautery was introduced, and greater attention was paid to cleanliness in operations. Simpler splints and braces were devised. The first description (by Guy de Chauliac, 1300-1368) of continuous traction using weights and pulleys for management of fractures originated during this period.

During the Renaissance (fifteenth to sixteenth centuries) attention was directed to the complete review of human anatomy based on actual dissection of the human body. Leonardo da Vinci's (1452-1519) contributions to the field of orthopaedics were significant. His artistic quest led him to illustrate virtually all muscles and joints, revealing the basic principles of stress and strain in muscle function. Attention during the Renaissance was directed toward the management of skeletal trauma, in part necessitated by many injuries occurring during wartime. The concept of field hospitals was introduced by the Spaniards during this period. Ambroise Paré (1510-1590) made many contributions to orthopaedics. He dealt extensively with fractures, including those of the vertebrae, resulting in cord compression. He introduced the operative approach to the vertebral column, which marked the beginning of modern spinal surgery. In 1536 he performed the first recorded joint excision of the elbow for a patient with destructive infection. The next joint resection was not attempted for two more centuries. His outstanding surgical contribution to orthopaedics was introducing the application of ligatures during amputation, which minimized hemorrhage and left the stump less painful and therefore more suitable for prosthetic wear.

The seventeenth century marked the beginning of orthopaedics as a medical specialty. During that century the Poor Relief Act (1610) was passed in England, focusing attention on the care of the crippled. Society became more aware of the unfortunate and was more considerate of the deformed and maimed (Bick, 1968).

During the eighteenth century Nicholas Andry contributed significantly to the repertoire of information, particularly the investigation of skeletal deformities. The specialty title, *orthopaedics*, came from the word *orthopaedia*, used as the title of a treatise published by Andry in 1741. He compounded the word *orthopaedia* from the words *orthos* (straight) and *paidios* (child) to express his belief that many musculoskeletal deformities begin in childhood. He proposed teaching different methods of preventing and correcting the deformities of children (Bick, 1968).

Procedures performed before the beginning of the nineteenth century were very simple and straight forward, including treatment of amputations, open fractures, and closed fractures. Orthopaedics came of age during the nineteenth and twentieth centuries. Diseases and disorders of the musculoskeletal system were explored. The first elective operation that could be called an orthopaedic procedure was a subcutaneous tenotomy first carried out by Delpech in 1816 and popularized by Stromeyer and Little 15 years later. The subcutaneous osteotomy followed. The introduction of anesthesia in 1847 permitted more extensive orthopaedic procedures. Until the introduction of antiseptic surgical precautions by Lister in 1865, however, such operations were accompanied by a substantial risk of infection.

In his book on operative surgery Theodor Kocher (1872-1917) developed the concept of approaching the deep anatomic structures by using the neutral zones between muscles, supplied by different nerves, to minimize damage (Kocher, 1911). Extensive studies of bone growth and repair were undertaken. Sir John Charnley (1911-1982) was recognized among twentieth-century orthopaedic surgeons for his initial contributions, including his writings on fracture healing, the closed treatment of fractures, and the principles of arthrodesis of joints using compressions. Subsequently a major contribution, the low-friction arthroplasty for hip arthritis, was developed by Charnley. He also emphasized the role of airborne bacterial wound contamination in the operating room and studied the influence of clean air systems in the setting (Evarts, 1990).

Modern orthopaedics has expanded from a narrow focus to apply to patients of all ages and now includes all congenital, traumatic, infectious, hereditary, metabolic, neoplastic, and degenerative processes to which the musculoskeletal system is subject. Many formerly prevalent diseases that affect the musculoskeletal system, including tuberculosis, poliomyelitis, tertiary syphilis, and rickets, have been decreased or controlled as a result of research in orthopaedics. Future developments will come from advances in immunology, microbiology, genetics, and microsurgery.

Fundamental advances in surgery have been dependent on the development of other branches of science and industry. These advances resulted, for example, in availability of the high-powered microscope and x-ray tube. Advances in the equipment used for procedures, such as power supplies, has improved patient outcomes. Orthopaedics has developed at a rapid pace, along with science and industry, to provide an intriguing, involved patient care opportunity.

As orthopaedics has developed as a surgical specialty, the nursing role of a specialist has evolved. The realm of orthopaedic patient populations and procedures requires the perioperative nurse to view orthopaedic surgery as a unique specialty, unlike other perioperative specialties, for the provision of quality care. The future of orthopaedic nursing is dependent on the extent of involvement undertaken by those caring for patients in this highly specialized area as changes continue. In a technical arena with a plenitude of equipment and the physical requirements of perioperative orthopaedics, nurses practicing in this area cannot lose sight of their role. Musculoskeletal conditions are a significant cause of restricted activity, lost wages, and increased health care costs. The ever-expanding body of knowledge related to the needs of individuals and families impacted by disorders of the musculoskeletal system has created an exciting opportunity for the nurse as a caregiver, consultant, educator, and researcher.

BIBLIOGRAPHY

Adams JC, Hamblen DL: *Outline of orthopaedics,* ed 11, Edinburgh, 1990, Churchill Livingstone, pp 1-4.

Bick EM: Primitive man and ancient practice. In *Source book of orthopaedics,* New York, 1968, Hafner.

Billings JS: History of surgery. In Dennis FS, editor: *System of surgery,* Philadelphia, 1895-1896, Lea Brothers.

Breasted JH: The Edwin Smith Papyrus, NY Historical Society, *Q Bull* 6:5, 1922.

Enneking WF: *Manual of orthopaedic surgery,* Chicago, 1979, American Orthopaedic Association.

Evarts MC: *Surgery of the musculoskeletal system,* ed 2, New York, 1990, Churchill Livingstone, pp 3-8.

Kocher T: *Text-book of operative surgery,* ed 3, New York, 1911, Macmillan, p 277.

LeVay D: *The history of orthopaedics,* New York, 1990, Panthenon Books.

McGinty JB and others: *Operative arthroscopy,* New York, 1991, Raven Press, pp 1-4.

Peltier LF: Historical perspectives of orthopaedic anatomy and surgical approaches. In Reckling FW, Reckling JB, Mohn MP, editors: *Orthopaedic anatomy and surgical approaches,* St Louis, 1990, Mosby.

2

The Orthopaedic Team

Teamwork is a requisite for efficiency in the perioperative setting, requiring trust and communication among those participating on the team. Direct teamwork includes communication among the physicians, their office personnel, and the perioperative nurse to determine specific procedural needs. Indirect teamwork includes understanding the preoperative and postoperative roles of the physical therapists or diagnosticians to be able to reinforce teaching. Preplanning, collaborative practice, and communication among health team members can facilitate a positive outcome (Walsh, 1991). Each team member has a responsibility to participate actively as a vital link, creating a team that provides the optimum patient care on the continuum.

PERIOPERATIVE ORTHOPAEDIC NURSE

The registered nurse specializing in perioperative nursing performs nursing activities in the preoperative, intraoperative, and postoperative phases of the patient's surgical experience (Association of Operating Room Nurses, 1992). Advances in technology and the expanding body of knowledge related to the needs of individuals and families impacted by disorders of the musculoskeletal system has caused much evolution in orthopaedic nursing. Orthopaedic nurses facilitate the promotion of wellness, self-care, and the prevention of illness and injury in individuals of all ages with degenerative, traumatic, inflammatory, neuromuscular, congenital, metabolic, and oncologic disorders. These specialized nurses practice in all health care settings, working independently and within an inter-disciplinary team. The nurse specializing in orthopaedics can facilitate a procedure by applying the nursing process and serving as a resource for the many procedures that take place in the specialty. The perioperative orthopaedic specialist has been challenged during recent years by developments in theoretic and clinical knowledge. This calls for a commitment to seeking educational opportunities and resources to practice effectively in this specialty. The "Scope of Orthopaedic Nursing Practice" (National Association of Orthopaedic Nurses, 1990) describes the beliefs, practice environment, practices, professional certification, and educational level of orthopaedic nurses and addresses issues relevant to the specialty.

The professional orthopaedic caregiver practices in collaboration with other health care professionals to provide appropriate, effective, and efficient health care. Orthopaedic nurses have a significant impact on the wellness of our society. The musculoskeletal conditions corrected during orthopaedic surgery can assist a patient in returning to normal levels of activity that previously would have resulted in pain and further illness. Procedures are performed on an outpatient and an inpatient basis, adding another dimension to the scope of orthopaedic perioperative practice. The phases of perioperative practice can be individualized to the setting, patient population, and surgical procedure to enhance the care of the orthopaedic patient. Nurses implementing the nursing process during each phase of care impact the outcome of the surgical procedure and promote wellness within society.

Challenges and expectations in the practice environment come not only from the expanding technology but also from the variety of health care consumers. The orthopaedic nurse cares for the pediatric, midlife, and elderly populations with both acute and chronic illnesses. The multiple needs of the consumer population provide the opportunity to practice perioperative nursing using a holistic approach.

ROLE OF THE ORTHOPAEDIC SURGEON

Surgical advances have changed the role of the orthopaedic surgeon. The equipment, supplies, instrumentation, and procedures change continually, resulting in a challenging practice environment. Surgeons have become highly specialized because of a need for individualized care and a demand for procedures within the specialty of orthopaedics, including joint reconstruction; sports medicine; oncologic orthopaedics; pediatric orthopaedics; hand, spine, and foot surgery; orthopaedic trauma; and general orthopaedics.

Surgeons have increased their reliance on other team members, creating a multidisciplinary environment and the unique opportunity for nurses to enhance patient care by practicing an expanded role. Working with physicians who have developed an expertise in one area allows the perioperative nurse to refine skills necessary to orchestrate the procedure.

REGISTERED NURSE FIRST ASSISTANT

The RN first assistant (RNFA) role encompasses a unique set of behaviors progressing on the skills continuum from basic competency to excellence (Association of Operating Room Nurses, 1990). Intraoperative responsibilities unique to the RNFA include:

- Handling tissue
- Providing exposure
- Using instruments
- Suturing
- Providing hemostasis

The RNFA role is a collaborative one, directly supervised by a surgeon and carried out to assist the surgeon in performing safe procedures with optimal results for the patient. The RNFA performs a single role and does not concurrently function as a scrub nurse.

The orthopaedic RNFA not only understands the surgical procedure, associated anatomy, and specific patient needs but also intraoperatively attends to the technical details of instrumentation, exposure, and principles of the procedures significant in the highly technical specialty of orthopaedics. Orthopaedic surgical procedures frequently require assistance in maintaining exposure of the surgical site, necessitating that the RNFA anticipate needs while holding extremities, applying traction, or maneuvering extremities. These activities, if managed appropriately, benefit the patient by allowing the physician to complete the procedure in a timely manner with minimal tissue trauma.

ANESTHESIA TEAM

Anesthesia care provided by the anesthesiologist or certified registered nurse anesthetist (CRNA) might also be specialized to orthopaedics. Patient risk and safety are always concerns during surgery and anesthesia, requiring vigilance and awareness of potential problems. The choice of anesthesia in orthopaedics is usually made by the anesthesiologist in consideration of the needs and preferences of the patient and surgeon.

Procedures require general and/or regional anesthesia or monitored anesthesia care. Nurses specializing in orthopaedics should be familiar with the methods of administration, medications used, and potential risks. Good communication between the anesthesia team and the nursing team enhances the care provided during the procedure and the patient outcome.

CERTIFIED SURGICAL TECHNOLOGIST

The surgical technologist complements activities of the registered nurse, the surgeon, and the anesthesia team. The technical skills required in orthopaedics can be supplemented by an individual who has an understanding of the procedures and needs of team members. The surgical technologist prepares and handles supplies and equipment, maintains a safe and therapeutic environment, and implements specific techniques and practices to assist in the perioperative setting (Atkinson, 1992). The surgical technologist's responsibilities include maintaining an aseptic environment and understanding surgical procedures and specialized instrument systems to meet the critical needs of orthopaedic patients.

OTHER PROVIDERS

Orthopaedic procedures require personnel in support positions that are nonnursing roles, working to meet the needs of the patient. These individuals may not be employees in the department or hospital but are a necessary link in the provision of satisfactory care. Support personnel include the radiologist, the radiology technician, product representatives, the physical therapist, and assistive support personnel.

Radiology Personnel

Many orthopaedic procedures require radiography immediately before, after, or during the procedure. The role of the radiologist is specialized and partially assumed by the physician during the procedure. The radiology technician plays a key support role in the operating room during many orthopaedic procedures requiring radiography (x-ray film or fluoroscopy) and must have an understanding of the expected outcome of the procedure. They must also have an understanding of asepsis and operating room sanitation to maintain cleanliness and sterility of the environment. A technician who can anticipate the surgical needs decreases the length of the procedure and frustration of the team members.

Product Representatives

The role of product representatives in orthopaedics has evolved during recent years. Hospitals cannot always purchase stock supplies of implants or equipment for infrequently scheduled procedures. The representative who maintains an awareness of the goals of the surgical department and hospital in addition to meeting the needs of the surgeon provides a beneficial patient care service. As new products become available on the market, it is also the responsibility of the registered nurse to be involved in product evaluation. The ability to communicate needs adequately with the product representative and to critique products objectively are public relations skills that benefit both the patients and the hospital.

Physical Therapist

The role of the physical therapist is not directly related to completing the orthopaedic procedure but does require an understanding of the preoperative therapeutic procedures or plan of care for adequate postoperative instruction. Some patients undergoing orthopaedic procedures may have received extensive physical therapy before deciding to pursue surgical intervention. Others must make a commitment to postoperative physical therapy to accomplish the desired outcome. The perioperative nurse specializing in orthopaedics can reinforce and strengthen the patient's understanding of the need for therapeutic interventions.

Assistive Support Personnel

Orthopaedic procedures benefit from knowledgeable support personnel working in the department. Procedures require physical strength to accomplish transferring, positioning, and preparing the patient. Care of the equipment and instruments is also necessary to meet intraoperative needs. The responsibilities applicable in other specialties may not apply in orthopaedics, resulting in the need for increasing the understanding of those responsible for assisting in the care of orthopaedic patients.

Individuals in different roles providing care for the orthopaedic patient have opportunities for collaborative perioperative nursing care. Collaboration requires an understanding of the common purpose of orthopaedic patient care, recognition of the unique skills provided by individuals providing the care, and communication of the patient's needs and care. An orthopaedic patient has special needs that can benefit from a collaborative approach by perioperative team members if the required time, energy, and commitment are invested in the process.

BIBLIOGRAPHY

Atkinson LJ: *Berry and Kohn's operating room technique,* ed 7, St Louis, 1992, Mosby.

Association of Operating Room Nurses: *Core curriculum for the RN first assistant,* Denver, 1990, AORN.

Association of Operating Room Nurses: *AORN standards and recommended practices for perioperative nursing—1992,* Denver, 1992, AORN.

Berg E: Progress in orthopedic surgery: the 1980's in review, *Orthop Nurs* 9:29, May/June 1990.

Groah L: *Operating room nursing, perioperative practice,* ed 2, Norwalk, 1990, Appleton & Lange.

Kneedler J, Dodge G: *Perioperative patient care, the nursing perspective,* Boston, 1983, Blackwell Scientific Publications.

Meeker M, Rothrock J: *Alexander's care of the patient in surgery,* ed 9, St Louis, 1991, Mosby.

National Association of Orthopaedic Nurses: Scope of orthopaedic nursing practice, *Orthop Nurs* 9:11, Nov/Dec 1990.

Walsh CR: Collaborative practice: a coordinated approach to patient care, *Orthop Nurs* 10:52, Sept/Oct 1991.

3

Musculoskeletal Structures

Two hundred six bones and their intervening cartilages make up the skeletal system and supporting framework of the body. Over 70% of the total body consists of joints, muscles, and associated ligaments, tendons, and bursae. The functions of the skeletal system are to:

- Support soft tissue of the body and provide form and shape
- Facilitate movement when overlying muscles contract
- Afford protection to the underlying organs of the body
- Produce blood cells (hematopoiesis)
- Store minerals for body use, especially calcium and phosphorus

TISSUE STRUCTURE

Bone is living tissue surrounded by soft tissue with vascular connections (Fig. 3-1). Bones share common features on gross examination. A dense layer of fibrous tissue, called periosteum, encloses the bone. Periosteum of children is thicker than that of adults, less adherent to bone, and more easily defined.

Periosteum is also incorporated into tendons and ligaments that are attached to bone. Another membrane, endosteum, lines the marrow cavities of the bones. It is a loosely woven vascular membrane that lines the medullary cavities. The two types of bone are cortical (compact) and cancellous (trabeculae). Both types have identical microscopic structures; the difference is in the relationship to the blood supply. Cancellous bone is soft, spongy bony tissue surrounded by blood vessels. It is located in flat, irregular short bones (vertebral bodies, diploe of cranial bones, sternum, ribs, pelvis, and iliac bones) and in the ends

of long bones (epiphyses). Cancellous bone consists of an interconnecting network of bone. Cortical bone is a thick ring surrounding a cavity containing bone marrow. It is found on the exterior portion of all bones and in the shaft (diaphysis) of long bones. It is dense and feels and looks like ivory.

Two types of marrow (Fig. 3-2) in the cavities of bones are forms of connective tissue containing numerous blood vessels. Yellow marrow fills the medullary cavities. It is composed mostly of fat cells and a few myelocytes. Red marrow (myeloid tissue) is found in cancellous bone. It contains immature red blood cells.

Bone is very vascular. Blood vessels in compact bone emerge from a large network of vessels in the periosteum. These vessels enter and leave the tissue through Volkmann's canals. The blood supply to the cancellous bone enters through the compact bone and runs through the cavities of the spongy bone (Fig. 3-3). At least one large nutrient artery enters the medullary cavity through a nutrient foramen (usually located at the center of the bone).

SKELETAL STRUCTURE

Bones are classified according to shape: long, short, flat, and irregular. Long bones (Fig. 3-4) are found in the extremities and consist of a diaphysis (shaft) with two expanded epiphyses (ends). Examples include the tibia, femur, and humerus. The ends are covered with articular (hyaline) cartilage, providing a surface for articulation and muscle attachment. They are curved to give more strength and are composed predominantly of compact bone. Short bones are cube shaped and consist mainly of spongy bone with a compact bone shell (e.g., carpal and tarsal bones). They are

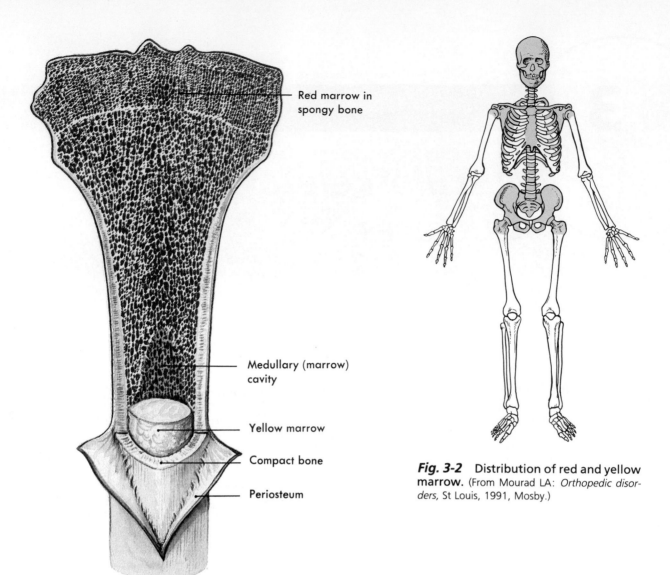

Fig. 3-1 Gross structure of long bone. (From Anthony CP, Thibodeau GA: *Textbook of anatomy and physiology,* ed 12, St Louis, 1987, Mosby.)

Red marrow in spongy bone

Medullary (marrow) cavity

Yellow marrow

Compact bone

Periosteum

Fig. 3-2 Distribution of red and yellow marrow. (From Mourad LA: *Orthopedic disorders,* St Louis, 1991, Mosby.)

Osteon (haversian system)

Circumferential lamellae

Blood vessels within haversian or central canal

Lacunae containing osteocytes

Canaliculi

Periosteum

Interstitial lamellae

Blood vessel within Volkmann's or perforating canal

Concentric lamellae

Fig. 3-3 Vascular structure of bone. (From Mourad LA: *Orthopedic disorders,* St Louis, 1991, Mosby.)

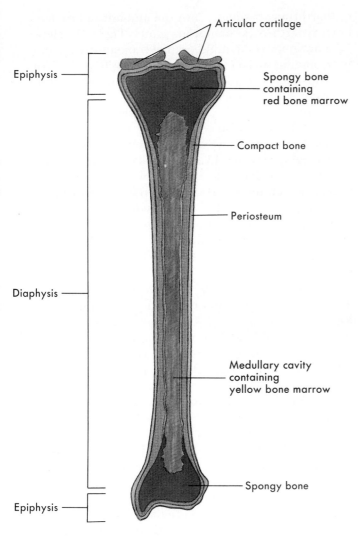

Articular cartilage

Epiphysis

Spongy bone containing red bone marrow

Compact bone

Periosteum

Diaphysis

Medullary cavity containing yellow bone marrow

Spongy bone

Epiphysis

Fig. 3-4 **Long-bone structure as seen in longitudinal section.** (From Anthony CP, Thibodeau GA: *Textbook of anatomy and physiology,* ed 12, St Louis, 1987, Mosby.)

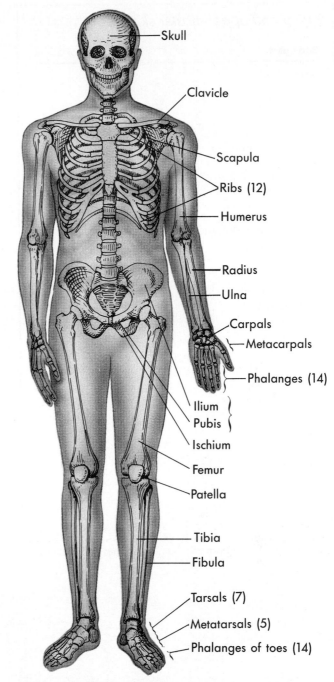

Skull

Clavicle

Scapula

Ribs (12)

Humerus

Radius

Ulna

Carpals

Metacarpals

Phalanges (14)

Ilium
Pubis
Ischium

Femur

Patella

Tibia

Fibula

Tarsals (7)

Metatarsals (5)

Phalanges of toes (14)

Fig. 3-5 **Skeletal structure.** (From Mourad LA: *Orthopedic disorders,* St Louis, 1991, Mosby.)

present where strength is needed but limited movement is required. Flat bones are thin and composed of two plates of compact bone with an intervening layer of cancellous bone (e.g., cranial bones, ribs, scapula, ilium). These bones give a great deal of protection and have large surface areas for muscle attachment.

Irregular bones are of various shapes and do not fit in the previous groups. The composition of these bones varies from mostly compact to a compact bony shell surrounding a cancellous bone center (e.g., some skull bones and vertebrae).

Other bones are not classified by shape. Sesamoid bones are free-floating bones usually found in tendons or joint capsules. The patella is the largest of these, but small ones are found in the tendons of the hands and feet. Wormian bones are small clusters of bones found between the joints of some cranial bones (e.g., parietal sutures). The skeletal structure is divided into axial and appendicular portions (Fig. 3-5). The ap-

pendicular division includes those bones forming the freely moving appendages of the upper and lower extremities and the bones of the shoulder and pelvic girdles. The axial skeleton consists of those bones found in the midline of the body. There are typically 80 bones in the axial skeleton and 126 bones in the appendicular division (see box on p. 12).

Joints are the junction between two or more bones. These are classified as synarthrotic, amphiarthrotic,

Axial and appendicular skeleton

Body part	Number of bones
Axial	
Skull	
Cranium	8
Face	14
Hyoid	1
Vertebral column	26
Thorax	
Ribs (12 pairs)	24
Sternum	1
Ossicles of the ear	6
Appendicular Skeleton	
Shoulder girdle	
Scapula	2
Clavicle	2
Upper extremity	
Humerus	2
Radius	2
Ulna	2
Carpus	16
Metacarpal bones	10
Phalanges	28
Pelvic girdle	
Innominate, coxa, hip	2
Lower extremity	
Femur	2
Tibia	2
Fibula	2
Patella	2
Tarsus	14
Metatarsals	10
Phalanges	28

From Hilt NE, Cogburn SB: *Manual of orthopedics*, St Louis, 1980, Mosby.

or diarthrotic, depending on the amount of articulation. Synarthroses, or fibrous joints (Fig. 3-6), allow little or no movement, do not have a joint cavity, and have binding surfaces of fibrous tissue or bone growth that do not allow movement. These can be syndesmoses or suture joints.

There are two amphiarthrotic, or slightly movable, types of joints, classified as synchondrosis or symphysis. Both types have cartilage between the bones. A synchondrosis has hyaline cartilage between two articulating surfaces, as in the epiphyseal plate between the epiphysis and the diaphysis. This cartilage is eventually replaced by bone. A symphysis has bone surfaces separated by fibrocartilage, as seen between vertebral bodies and at the pubic symphysis. The fibrocartilage remains throughout life and is not replaced by bone.

Diarthroses are freely movable joints (Fig. 3-7). They are the body's most mobile and most numerous joints and have a complex structure (Fig. 3-8). They are surrounded by a fibrous joint capsule and are lined on all but the articular surfaces with an epithelium called synovium. Synovial fluid, rich in hyaluronic acid, is highly polymerized, which accounts for its nourishing and lubricating qualities. Protein, fat, monocytes, macrophages, and other blood leukocytes are found in synovial fluid. Synovial fluid bathes the joint to reduce friction of the articulating surfaces. The articular surfaces of the bones forming the joint are covered with articular cartilage. The joint may be divided by an articular disk or meniscus, the periphery of which is continuous with the fibrous capsule, while its free surfaces are covered with synovium. Bursae

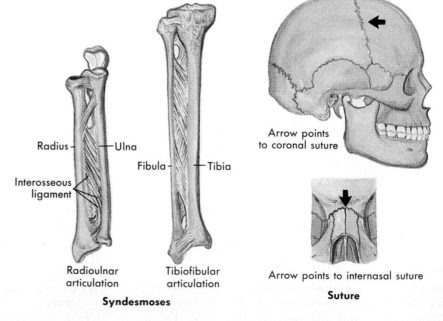

Fig. 3-6 Synarthrotic (fibrous) joints. (From Thibodeau GA, Patton KT: *Anatomy and physiology,* ed 2, St Louis, 1993, Mosby.)

Radius — Ulna

Interosseous ligament

Radioulnar articulation

Fibula — Tibia

Tibiofibular articulation

Syndesmoses

Arrow points to coronal suture

Arrow points to internasal suture

Suture

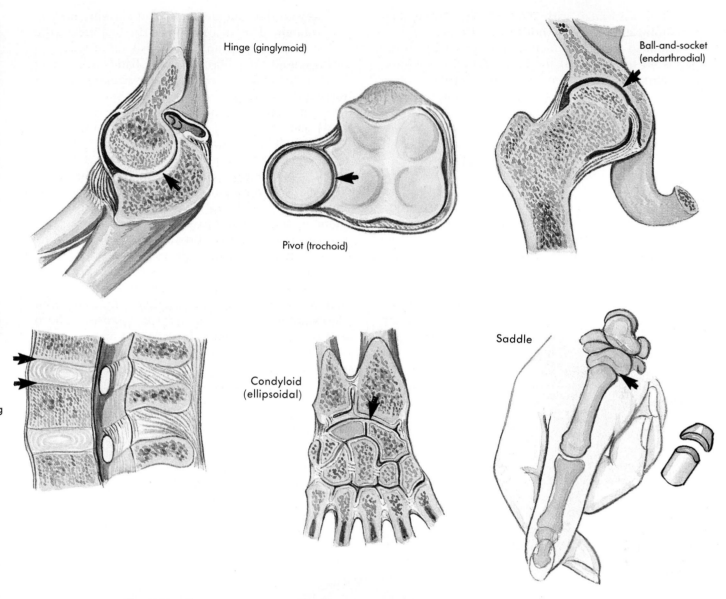

Hinge (ginglymoid)

Pivot (trochoid)

Ball-and-socket (endarthrodial)

Condyloid (ellipsoidal)

Saddle

Fig. 3-7   Diarthrotic joints. (From Thibodeau GA: *Anthony's textbook of anatomy and physiology,* ed 13, St Louis, 1990, Mosby.)

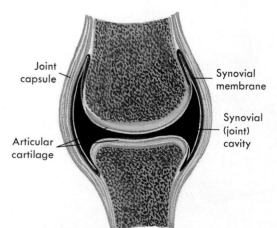

Joint capsule

Synovial membrane

Synovial (joint) cavity

Articular cartilage

Fig. 3-8   Structure of a diarthrotic joint. (From Anthony CP, Thibodeau GA: *Textbook of anatomy and physiology,* ed 13, St Louis, 1990, Mosby.)

are often associated with synovial joints, sometimes communicating directly with the joint space.

The degree of movement at the synovial joint depends on the shape of the bones forming the joint, the tautness of the ligaments of the capsule, and the position and action of muscles whose tendons cross or enter the joint. Types of diarthrotic joints include:

- Ginglymoid, or hinge. One surface is concave, and one surface is convex. Movement is generally flexion or extension. Examples are the knee, the radial and humeral bones of the elbow, and the ankle.
- Trochoid, or pivot. An articulating surface rotates around a peg or projection, and movement is rotation on one axis. Examples include rotation of the atlas on the axis and proximal articulation of the radius on the ulna.
- Enarthrodial, or ball-and-socket. The head fits in a concave socket, allowing for the most movement. Flexion, extension, and circumduction are the three planes of movement allowed. Examples are the hip and shoulder joints.
- Arthrodial, or gliding. Articular surfaces are flat in the joint, with no axis of movement. The sacrum, the ilium, and many of the carpal bones form this type of joint.
- Ellipsoidal, or condyloid. An oval condyle fits into an elliptic cavity. Movement is in two planes that are perpendicular to each other. Extension, flexion, adduction, abduction, and circumduction are allowed, as in the movement of the radius on the carpal bones.
- Saddle. The bone fits onto a convex surface of another bone, allowing for the same movements

as with the condyloid joint but allowing no axial rotation. The articulation of the first metacarpal with the trapezium forms this kind of joint.

Ligaments are fibrous tissue bands connecting bone to bone. They create greater strength by reinforcing the anatomic area. Ligaments such as the medial or lateral collateral ligaments of the knee blend in the joint capsule by joining bone ends together.

The **skull** is composed of 22 bones and rests on the cranial end of the vertebral column (Fig. 3-9). The cranial bones enclose and protect the brain. These bones are of greatest importance in orthopaedics because many muscles of the neck and back attach to them at some point. Orthopaedic procedures rarely involve cranial and facial structures.

The **vertebral column** forms the flexible longitudinal axis of the skeleton (Fig. 3-10). It is composed of a series of bones called vertebrae and is approximately 28 inches long in the adult. The column encloses and protects the spinal cord, supports the head, and provides attachment for ribs and muscles of the back. Intervertebral foramina are openings between the vertebrae that allow for passage of spinal nerves from the cord. There are 7 cervical vertebrae, 12 thoracic vertebrae, 5 lumbar vertebrae, 1 sacral vertebra (formed by the fusion of 5 vertebrae), and 1 or 2 coccygeal vertebrae (formed by the fusion of 4 or 5 vertebrae). The vertebrae are separated from each other by intervertebral disks (Fig. 3-11). These disks consist of cartilaginous end plates, a fibrocartilaginous outer ring (annulus fibrosus), and a gelatinous center (nucleus pulposus). They increase the strength and pliability of the intervertebral joints. The ligaments joining the disks are extensive; these include the

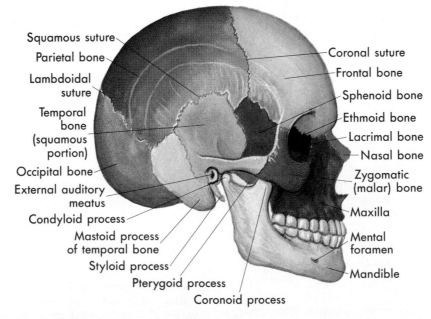

Fig. 3-9   Skull viewed from right side. (From Thibodeau GA, Patton KT: *Anatomy and physiology,* ed 2, St Louis, 1993, Mosby.)

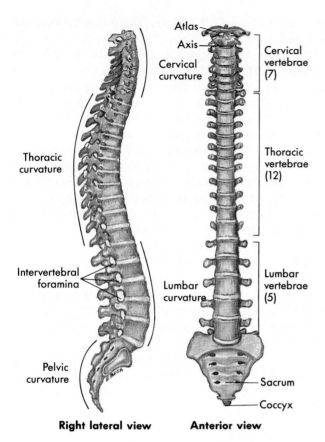

Right lateral view   **Anterior view**

Fig. 3-10   Vertebral column. (From Thibodeau GA, Patton KT: *Anatomy and physiology*, ed 12, St Louis, 1993, Mosby.)

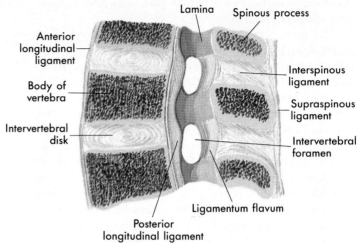

Fig. 3-11   Sagittal section of lumbar vertebrae and ligaments. (From Thibodeau GA, Patton KT: *Anatomy and physiology*, ed 2, St Louis, 1993, Mosby.)

ligamenta flava, located on the roof of the intervetebral foramen.

Viewed laterally, there are four alternately concave and convex curves in the spinal column. These curves increase the column strength, absorb shocks, maintain balance and position, and protect the column from fracture. Three conditions that involve exaggerated curvature of the column are scoliosis, left-to-right curvature, kyphosis, exaggerated anterior concavity (hunchback); and lordosis, exaggerated lumbar curvature (swayback).

All vertebrae of the spinal column have similar structures, with different shapes, sizes, and articular surfaces. A typical vertebra has a thick, anteriorly located, spherical body to confer weight-bearing ability (Fig. 3-12). The superior and inferior surfaces of the body are roughened by the attachment of the intervertebral disks. Extending posteriorly from the body is a neural arch composed of bilateral pedicles united posteriorly by a lamina of bone. These structures surround the vertebral foramen, forming the vertebral canal for passage of the spinal column. Processes found on the neural arch include bilateral, transverse,

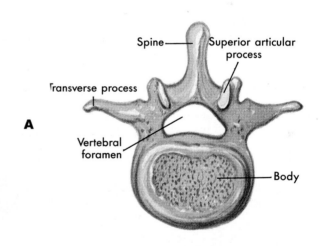

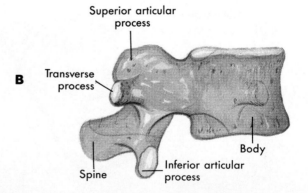

Fig. 3-12   Third lumbar vertebra. **A,** Superior view. **B,** Lateral view. (From Thibodeau GA, Patton KT: *Anatomy and physiology*, ed 2, St Louis, 1993, Mosby.)

superior, and inferior articular processes and a single spinous process.

The seven cervical vertebrae have smaller bodies and larger arches than the thoracic vertebrae. Vertebrae C2 through C6 have a bifid spinous process, and all of the cervical vertebrae have transverse foramina in the transverse processes that allow for passage of the vertebral arteries, veins, and nerves. The first cervical vertebra, the atlas, supports the head. It is circular, without a body or spinous process. Its superior articular processes articulate with the occipital condyles, which permits nodding of the head. The inferior articular processes articulate with the second cervical vertebra, the axis. This vertebra has a body with an upward projection, called the dens or odontoid process, which articulates through the atlas ring, forming a pivot joint that allows side-to-side movement. Vertebrae C3 through C6 fit the typical description of the vertebrae. Vertebra C7 is similar in shape and form except that its spinous process is not bifid and it can be palpated at the base of the neck.

The 12 thoracic vertebrae have bodies that are heavier, and their transverse processes are longer. Their spinous processes project downward, and all but vertebrae T11 and T12 have facets for articulation with the ribs.

The five lumbar vertebrae are the largest and strongest of the vertebrae, and their spinous processes are heavy and blunt. Their superior articular processes project medially instead of superiorly, and the inferior articular processes are directed laterally instead of inferiorly. The placement of these processes stabilizes the articulations of the lumbar vertebrae.

The sacrum, formed by the fusion of five vertebrae, is the foundation of the pelvic girdle. It is concave anteriorly and placed posteriorly between the two coxae, or hip bones. Anteriorly, four transverse lines indicating where fusion has occurred are visible, as are four pairs of pelvic foramina. On the dorsal aspect of the sacrum are medial and lateral sacral crests and four pairs of dorsal foramina. An extension of the vertebral canal, the sacral canal, extends into the sacrum. The coccyx, formed by the fusion of four or five vertebrae, articulates with the sacrum and is a vestige of a tail.

The **thorax,** or chest, is supported by a bony cage composed of the ribs, sternum, costal cartilages, and thoracic vertebral bodies (Fig. 3-13). It is narrow su-

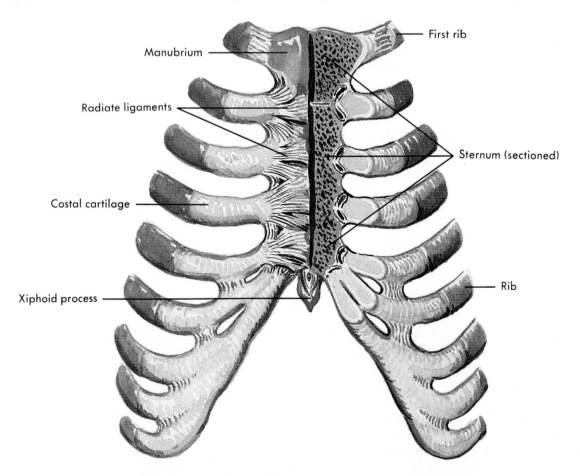

Fig. 3-13 Thorax, anterior view. (From Thibodeau GA: *Anthony's textbook of anatomy and physiology,* ed 13, St Louis, 1990, Mosby.)

periorly and wide inferiorly. It encloses and protects the organs of the thoracic cavity and supports the bony structure of the shoulder girdle and upper extremity.

The sternum is about 6 inches long and forms the medial part of the anterior thoracic wall. It is composed of three fused parts: a superior triangular manubrium, which articulates with the clavicle and the first two ribs; a middle piece, the body of which articulates with ribs 2 through 10; and an inferior xiphoid process that has no rib attachment but does give abdominal muscle attachment.

There are 12 pairs of ribs, which increase in length from 1 through 7 and decrease in length from 8 through 12. Ribs 1 through 7 attach directly to the sternum by means of costal cartilage and are called true ribs. Ribs 8 through 12 do not attach to the sternum and are called false ribs. Ribs 8 through 10 attach to each other by means of adjoining cartilage and then attach to the seventh costal cartilage. Ribs 11 and 12 do not attach to those above them and thus are considered floating ribs. The head of each rib articulates posteriorly with a facet on a vertebral body. Ribs 2 through 9 articulate with the bodies of two adjacent vertebrae. Ribs 1 and 10 through 12 articulate only with their respective vertebral bodies. Ribs 11 and 12

have no articulations with vertebral tubercles or transverse processes.

Each **shoulder girdle** consists of the clavicle and scapula. The two shoulder girdles act as the points of attachment of the upper extremities to the axial skeleton. These girdles have no articulation with the vertebral column. The clavicle, or collarbone, forms the anterior portion of the girdle, holding it away from the chest wall. It articulates in the anterior midline with the manubrium of the sternum and laterally with the acromion process of the scapula, forming the acromioclavicular joint. A conoid tubercle is found on the inferior surface of the lateral end of the clavicle and serves as attachment for a ligament.

The scapula, or shoulder blade (Fig. 3-14), is a large, flat, triangular bone located at the level between the second and seventh ribs in the dorsal part of the thorax. A sharp projection crosses diagonally on the upper third of the posterior surface of the flat body of the bone. The lateral extension of the spine is the acromion process, which articulates with the clavicle. Below the acromion is the glenoid cavity, which forms a socket for the head of the humerus. At the lateral end of the superior border is an anterior projection, the coracoid process, which serves for muscle attach-

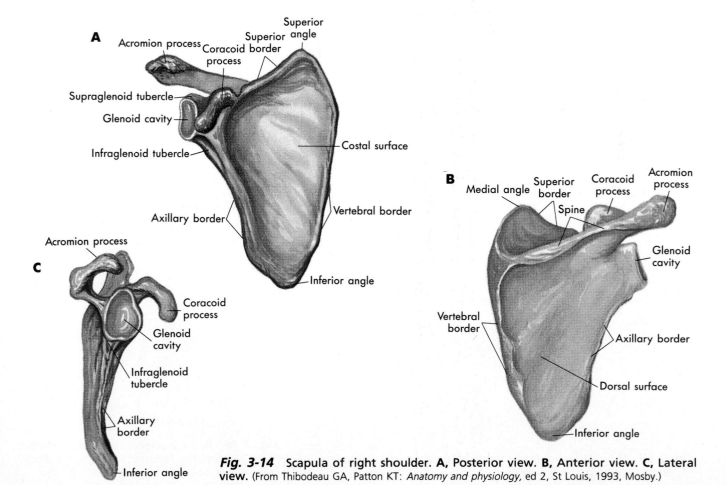

Fig. 3-14 Scapula of right shoulder. **A,** Posterior view. **B,** Anterior view. **C,** Lateral view. (From Thibodeau GA, Patton KT: *Anatomy and physiology,* ed 2, St Louis, 1993, Mosby.)

ment. The supraspinous, infraspinous, teres minor, and subscapular muscles stabilize the shoulder joint (Fig. 3-15); these make up the rotator cuff.

The acromioclavicular joint is the articulating structure between the outer end of the clavicle and the articular facet on the inner border of the acromion. The shoulder joint is a ball-and-socket joint formed by the head of the humerus and a shallow glenoid cavity. The joint is surrounded by a loose capsule to allow three planes of motion.

The **upper extremity** consists of the bones of the upper arm, lower arm, wrist, and hand. The humerus, or upper arm bone, is composed of a shaft and two ends (Fig. 3-16). It articulates as a ball-and-socket joint formed by the rounded head within the glenoid cavity of the scapula. Just below the head is a groove called the anatomic neck, the area of attachment to the capsule of the shoulder joint. The greater tubercle is a lateral projection below the neck, with impressions for insertion of the supraspinous, infraspinous, and teres minor tendons. The lesser tubercle is an anterior projection just below the neck, with an impression for insertion of the tendon of the subscapular muscle. An intertubercular groove for passage of the tendon of the biceps muscle is between the two tubercles. Below these tubercles the humerus narrows into a surgical neck, an area frequently requiring treatment for humeral fracture. At the deltoid tuberosity on the shaft, the humerus begins to flatten into a broad distal end. On the posterior surface of the shaft is the radial groove, through which the radial nerve passes. There are two projections from the medial and lateral margins of the lower end of the humerus: the medial and lateral epicondyles. The lower end of the humerus

has two flattened areas: a lateral capitellum that articulates with the radius and a medial trochlea that articulates with the ulna. Above the capitellum is the radial fossa, which receives the head of the radius when the forearm is flexed. Above the trochlea, on the anterior surface of the humerus, is a depression, the coronoid fossa, which receives the coronoid process of the ulna when it flexes onto the humerus. On the posterior end of the humerus is the olecranon fossa, which receives the olecranon process of the ulna when it is extended.

The radius and ulna are the bones of the forearm (Fig. 3-17). The radius is the bone of the forearm on the thumb side. The head, located proximally, articulates with the capitellum of the humerus and the radial notch of the ulna. The biceps muscle attaches on the medial aspect in the radial tuberosity. The ellipsoidal, or condyloid, joint allows movement of the radius on the carpal bones. The distal end of the radius has an ulnar notch for articulation with the ulna and the styloid process. The broadened distal end of the radius articulates with the lunate and scaphoid bones of the wrist.

The ulna is the medially placed bone of the forearm. The olecranon processes at the proximal end can be palpated at the elbow. The smooth area between

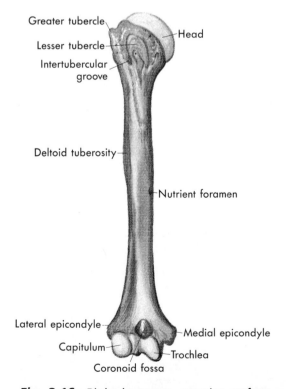

Fig. 3-16 Right humerus, anterior surface. (From Thibodeau GA, Patton KT: *Anatomy and physiology*, ed 2, St Louis, 1993, Mosby.)

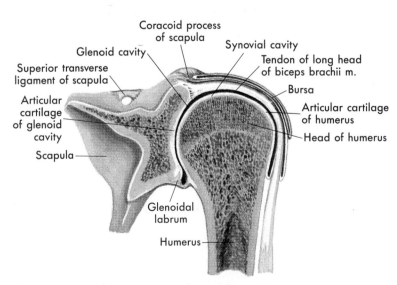

Fig. 3-15 Shoulder joint as viewed from behind. (From Thibodeau GA, Patton KT: *Anatomy and physiology*, ed 2, St Louis, 1993, Mosby.)

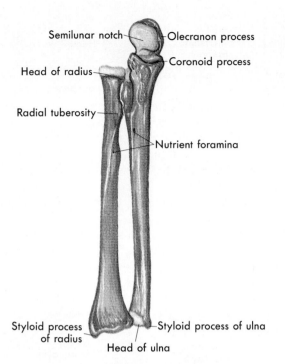

Semilunar notch — Olecranon process
— Coronoid process
Head of radius —
Radial tuberosity —
— Nutrient foramina
Styloid process of radius — Styloid process of ulna
Head of ulna

Fig. 3-17 **Right radius and ulna, anterior surface.** (From Thibodeau GA, Patton KT: *Anatomy and physiology*, ed 2, St Louis, 1993, Mosby.)

these two olecranon processes is the trochlear notch, which articulates with the trochlea of the humerus. The head of the ulna is at its distal end, and from it extends a projection, the styloid process, which is palpable at the wrist.

The carpus, or wrist, is composed of two transverse rows of small carpal bones (Fig. 3-18). In the dorsal anatomic position the distal row of bones contains the hamate, capitate, trapezoid, and trapezium bones. This distal row articulates with the bones that constitute the palm of the hand, including the scaphoid, lunate, triquetrum, and pisiform. The scaphoid serves as a link to stabilize and coordinate movement. Wrist bones are dependent on ligaments for movement, since muscles and tendons are not attached to these bones. Each of the five metacarpals situated in the palm consists of a proximal base, a shaft, and a distal head. The metacarpals are numbered from 1 to 5 beginning at the thumb, or lateral side. The heads articulate with the proximal phalanges of each finger. Each digit except the thumb has a proximal, middle, and distal phalanx, totaling 14 phalanges on each hand. The thumb has only two: one proximal and one distal.

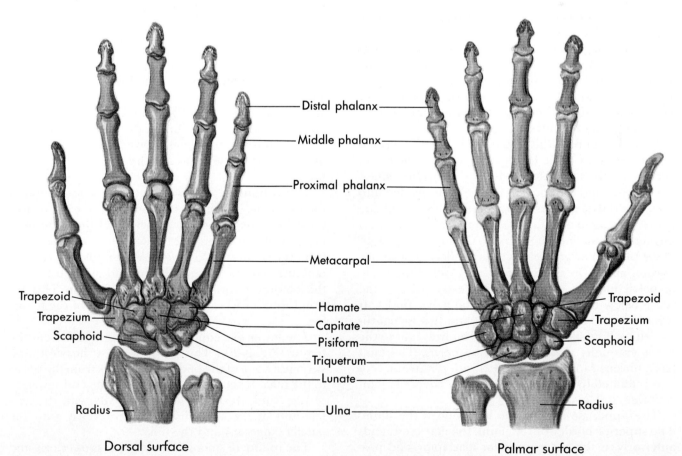

Distal phalanx
Middle phalanx
Proximal phalanx
Metacarpal
Trapezoid — Hamate — Trapezoid
Trapezium — Capitate — Trapezium
Scaphoid — Pisiform — Scaphoid
Triquetrum
Lunate
Radius — Ulna — Radius

Dorsal surface   Palmar surface

Fig. 3-18 **Right hand and wrist.** (From Thibodeau GA, Patton KT: *Anatomy and physiology*, ed 2, St Louis, 1993, Mosby.)

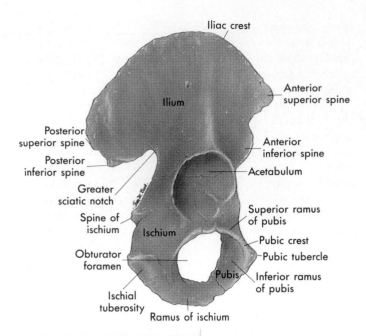

Fig. 3-19 Hip bone disarticulated to view internal surface and acetabulum. (From Thibodeau GA, Patton KT: *Anatomy and physiology,* ed 2, St Louis, 1993, Mosby.)

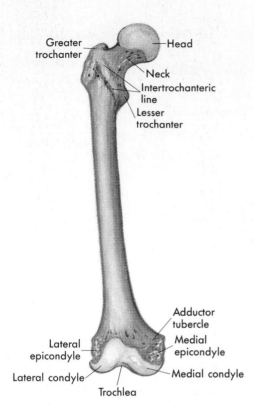

Fig. 3-20 Right femur, anterior surface. (From Thibodeau GA, Patton KT: *Anatomy and physiology,* ed 2, St Louis, 1993, Mosby.)

The **lower extremity** consists of bones of the hip, thigh, lower leg, ankle, and foot.

The **pelvic girdle** is composed of two coxae, or hip bones. These two bones unite anteriorly at the pubic symphysis, and posteriorly both attach to the lateral aspect of the sacrum. The pelvic girdle functions to support and stabilize the lower extremities and protect the organs that lie in the pelvis.

Each innominate (hip) bone (Fig. 3-19) is formed by the fusion of three bones: the ischium, the ilium, and the pubis. The pelvis includes the two hip bones, the sacrum, and the coccyx. The pelvis is divided into a greater (false) and lesser (true) pelvis by an oblique plane passing from the prominence of the sacrum through the pectineal lines and to the superior margin of the pubis. The greater pelvis is the flaring posterior portion above the narrow bony ring called the brim, or pelvic inlet, of the pelvis. The lesser pelvis is the space below the pelvic brim and the pelvic outlet. It is bound by the tip of the coccyx and two ischial tuberosities. The sacroiliac transmits body weight to the lower extremity through the bony pelvis. The joint has a fibrous capsule and is lined with synovium. Motion is limited by strong ligaments that cover the joint capsule.

The upper portion of the hip bone is the ilium. The superior border of the ilium, the iliac crest, ends anteriorly as the anterosuperior iliac spine and posteriorly as the posterosuperior iliac spine. The inner surface of the ilium is the iliac fossa, where muscles attach, and posterior to the fossa is the iliac tuberosity, at which the sacroiliac ligament attaches. The outer (lateral) surface of the wing of the ilium is marked by three distinct gluteal lines—posterior, anterior, and inferior—which serve as attachments for the gluteal muscles.

The ischium is the lowest and strongest portion of the hip bone. The ramus of the ischium extends forward from the tuberosity and body of the ischium to unite with the pubis. This surrounds a large aperture, the obturator foramen. At the point of the lateral fusion of the ilium, ischium, and pubis just above the obturator foramen is the acetabulum. This fusion forms a socket into which the head of the femur fits.

The lower extremity receives its support from the femur (Fig. 3-20). This is the longest, heaviest, and strongest bone of the body and extends from the pelvis to the tibia. It receives and supports the entire weight of the trunk. It articulates proximally with the acetabulum of the coxal bone and inferiorly with the patella (kneecap) and the tibia.

The rounded, smooth head projects superiorly and medially for articulation with the hip bone in a ball-

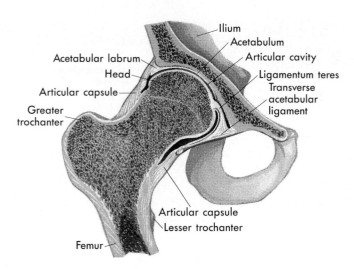

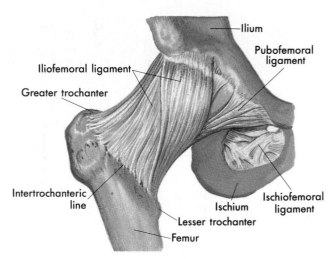

Fig. 3-21 Hip joint, frontal section. (From Thibodeau GA, Patton KT: *Anatomy and physiology*, ed 2, St Louis, 1993, Mosby.)

Fig. 3-22 Hip joint, anterior view. (From Thibodeau GA, Patton KT: *Anatomy and physiology*, ed 2, St Louis, 1993, Mosby.)

and-socket joint (Fig. 3-21). The socket is deep in the anteroposterior direction and is deepened further by a fibrocartilaginous rim, the glenoid labrum. This rim stabilizes the position of the femur. The labrum is incomplete inferiorly, but is held together by a transverse ligament. A Y-shaped iliofemoral ligament strengthens the joint anteriorly and prevents hyperextension (Fig. 3-22). The intracapsular ligamentum teres loosely attaches the head of the femur at the fovea capitis. The proximal end of the femur consists of a constricted neck and upper portion of the shaft. At the top of the shaft on the posterior aspect are the greater trochanter, consisting of cancellous bone, and the lesser trochanter. The greater trochanter serves as the point of insertion of the abductor and external rotator muscles. The lesser trochanter is the point of insertion for the iliopsoas muscle. Between the trochanters is an anterior intertrochanteric line and a posterior intertrochanteric crest. The shaft of the femur curves, directing the distal end more medially. A roughened vertical ridge, the linea aspera femoris, runs down the posterior surface of the shaft.

Distally the shaft broadens into rounded, smooth medial and lateral condyles, which articulate with the tibia. Above the condyles are roughened medial and lateral epicondyles. The condylar surfaces expand anteriorly in the midline to form an articular surface for the patella, the intercondylar or patellar groove. Above the medial epicondyle is the adductor tubercle, and on the posterior surface between the condyles is the intercondylar fossa, which receives the intercondylar eminence of the tibia when it flexes onto the femur.

The tibia and fibula form the lower leg (Fig. 3-23). The tibia, or shinbone, is the larger and more medially

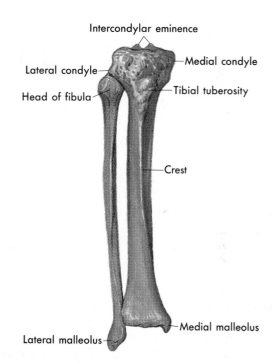

Fig. 3-23 Right tibia and fibula, anterior surface. (From Thibodeau GA, Patton KT: *Anatomy and physiology*, ed 2, St Louis, 1993, Mosby.)

placed bone of the lower leg. It articulates proximally with the femur and fibula and distally with the fibula and talus. On the proximal end of the tibia are smooth, concave, medial, and lateral condyles that articulate with the condyles of the femur (Fig. 3-24). Between the condyles is the intercondylar eminence, which projects upward. Anterior and posterior to the eminence is the intercondylar fossa. On the anterosuperior surface below the condyles is a raised, roughened

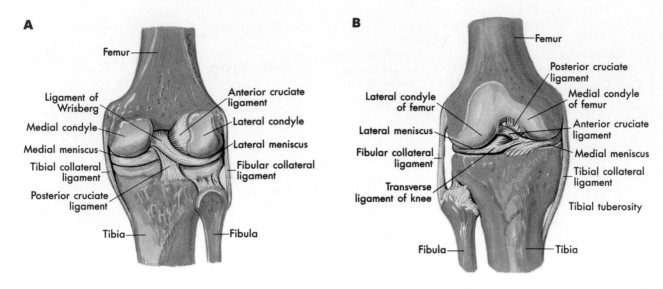

Fig. 3-24 Right knee joint. **A,** Anterior view. **B,** Posterior view. (From Thibodeau GA, Patton KT: *Anatomy and physiology,* ed 2, St Louis, 1993, Mosby.)

tibial tuberosity. Below the tuberosity the shaft narrows and a sharp anterior margin can be felt through the skin. The posterosuperior border has a prominent popliteal line, and below this line the posterior surface of the shaft flattens out. The distal end of the tibia is extended medially as the medial malleolus and notched laterally as the fibular notch for articulation with the fibula.

The fibula is a long, narrow bone lateral to the tibia. Its proximal expanded head articulates with the tibia. Its distal end extends as the lateral malleolus, which articulates with the talus as a ginglymoid, or hinge,

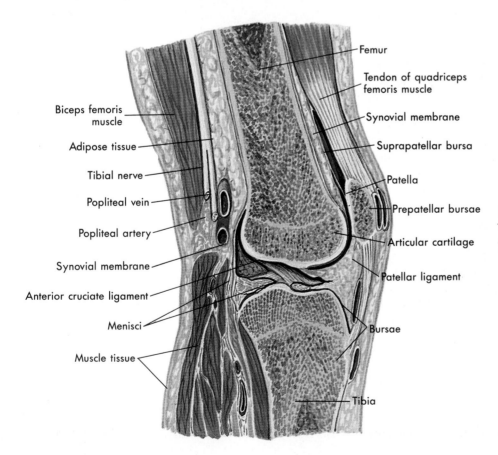

Fig. 3-25 Knee joint, sagittal section. (From Thibodeau GA, Patton KT: *Anatomy and physiology,* ed 2, St Louis, 1993, Mosby.)

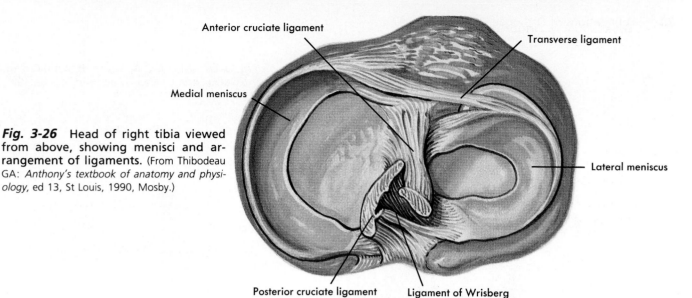

Fig. 3-26 Head of right tibia viewed from above, showing menisci and arrangement of ligaments. (From Thibodeau GA: *Anthony's textbook of anatomy and physiology*, ed 13, St Louis, 1990, Mosby.)

Anterior cruciate ligament

Transverse ligament

Medial meniscus

Lateral meniscus

Posterior cruciate ligament

Ligament of Wrisberg

joint. The lower medial portion of the fibula also articulates with the fibular notch of the tibia.

Anteriorly the tendon of the quadriceps femoris covers the joint and attaches to the patella, the patellar ligament, and then to the tibial tuberosity (Fig. 3-25). The patella, or kneecap, is a triangular sesamoid bone found on the anterior aspect of the knee joint embedded in the tendon of the quadriceps femoris muscle. The broad base is located superiorly; the apex points inferiorly. The patella articulates with the condyles of the femur but not with the tibia. The patella is held in position by ligaments and muscles and is surrounded by bursae. The knee joint, a diarthrotic joint, allows flexion and extension but also allows some gliding movement as the joint approaches complete extension or the locked position. The medial tibial collateral ligament, extending from the medial epicondyle of the femur to the medial condyle of the tibia, gives strength to the medial aspect of the joint. Laterally the fibular collateral ligament passes from the lateral femoral epicondyle to the head of the fibula.

Anteroposterior support of the joint is provided by the cruciate ligament (Fig. 3-26). The anterior cruciate ligament (ACL) passes from the intercondylar eminence of the tibia to the medial surface of the lateral femoral condyle. The posterior cruciate ligament (PCL) extends from the posterior portion of the intercondyloid fossa of the tibia to the posterior part of the lateral meniscus and the medial femoral condyle. A fold of synovial membrane covers both cruciate ligaments on their front and side. Posteriorly the PCL blends with the joint capsule.

The knee joint has two articular disks, or menisci, between the articular surfaces of the femur and tibia. These medial and lateral menisci are wedge-shaped crescents of fibrocartilage. The thick outer edges are attached to the fibrous joint capsule, and the thin inner edges are unattached. The function of the menisci

is to provide lateral support to the joint, distribute weight load across the knee joint, and promote capsular stability. The inside of the joint capsule is lined with synovial membrane, which secretes synovial fluid. The synovium does not cover the articular hyaline cartilage but does bathe the menisci. The synovial fluid of this joint prevents extreme wear and tear.

The bones of the foot (Fig. 3-27) include the tarsals, metatarsals, and phalanges, forming three arches: the medial longitudinal arch, the lateral longitudinal arch, and the transverse arch. The medial longitudinal arch comprises the talus, the navicular bone, three cunei-

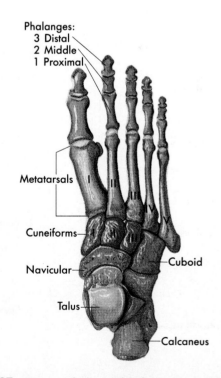

Phalanges:
3 Distal
2 Middle
1 Proximal

Metatarsals

Cuneiforms

Navicular

Talus

Cuboid

Calcaneus

Fig. 3-27 Bones of the right foot. (From Thibodeau GA, Patton KT: *Anatomy and physiology*, ed 2, St Louis, 1993, Mosby.)

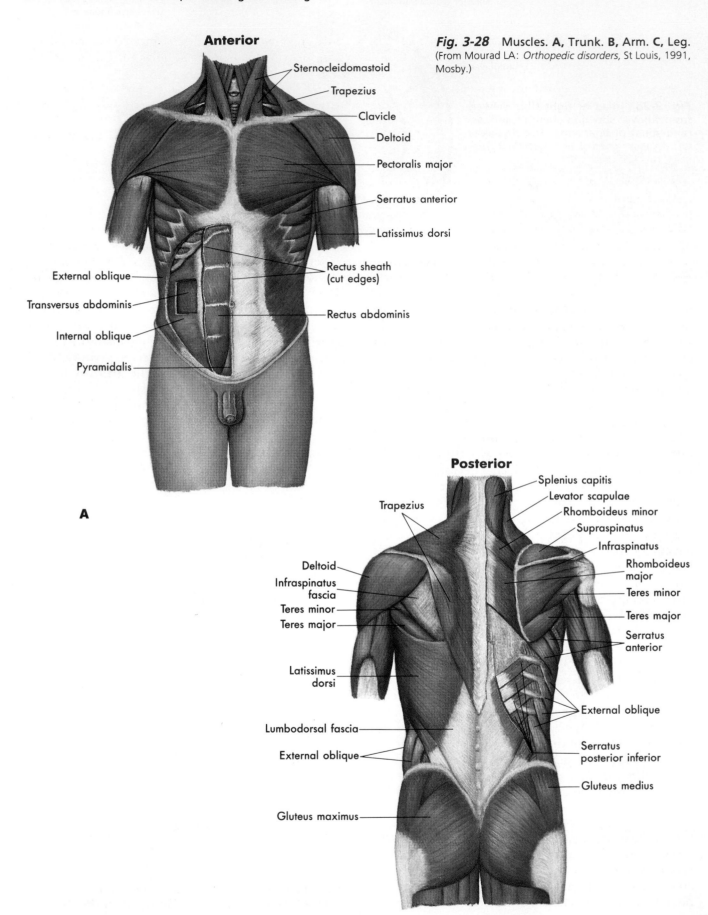

Anterior

Sternocleidomastoid

Trapezius

Clavicle

Deltoid

Pectoralis major

Serratus anterior

Latissimus dorsi

Rectus sheath
(cut edges)

External oblique

Transversus abdominis

Internal oblique

Rectus abdominis

Pyramidalis

A

Fig. 3-28 Muscles. **A,** Trunk. **B,** Arm. **C,** Leg.
(From Mourad LA: *Orthopedic disorders,* St Louis, 1991,
Mosby.)

Posterior

Splenius capitis

Levator scapulae

Rhomboideus minor

Supraspinatus

Infraspinatus

Rhomboideus
major

Teres minor

Teres major

Serratus
anterior

Trapezius

Deltoid

Infraspinatus
fascia

Teres minor

Teres major

Latissimus
dorsi

Lumbodorsal fascia

External oblique

External oblique

Serratus
posterior inferior

Gluteus medius

Gluteus maximus

form bones, and the first three metatarsal bones. The lateral longitudinal arch consists of the calcaneum, the cuboid, and metatarsal bones 4 and 5. The transverse arch includes the bases of the metatarsal bones, the cuboid, and three cuneiform bones. The arches have several functions, including distributing the weight of the body over the entire foot, providing rigidity and strength to the foot as a lever, providing a protected space for the vessels and nerves of the sole of the foot, and providing a resilient spring for shock absorption.

Of the seven tarsals, the talus is most superior, articulating superiorly with the fibula and tibia and inferiorly with the largest tarsal bone: the calcaneus, or heel bone. The talus bears the body weight and transmits a large portion of it to the calcaneus and the remainder to the anterior tarsals. The neck of the talus holds the strong interosseous talocalcaneal ligament. The posterior surface of the talus forms a groove for the flexor hallucis longus tendon. The navicular bone, cuneiform bones, and cuboid bone are held together by a ligamentous network. A groove on the plantar surface of the cuboid bone holds the tendon of peroneus longus.

The metatarsal bones are numbered 1 through 5 from the medial to the lateral aspect of the foot. Digits 2 through 5 have proximal, middle and, distal phalanges, whereas the great toe, or digit 1, has only proximal and distal phalanges.

MUSCULAR STRUCTURE

Within the body there are three varieties of muscle: smooth muscle, cardiac muscle, and skeletal muscle (Fig. 3-28). Skeletal muscle constitutes over one third of the total body mass. Muscle forms include flat and sheetlike, short and thick, and long and slender muscles. Muscle fibers have the ability to shorten to almost one half their resting length; therefore the length of each muscle is proportional to the distance it is required to contract. Each fiber of muscle has a delicate

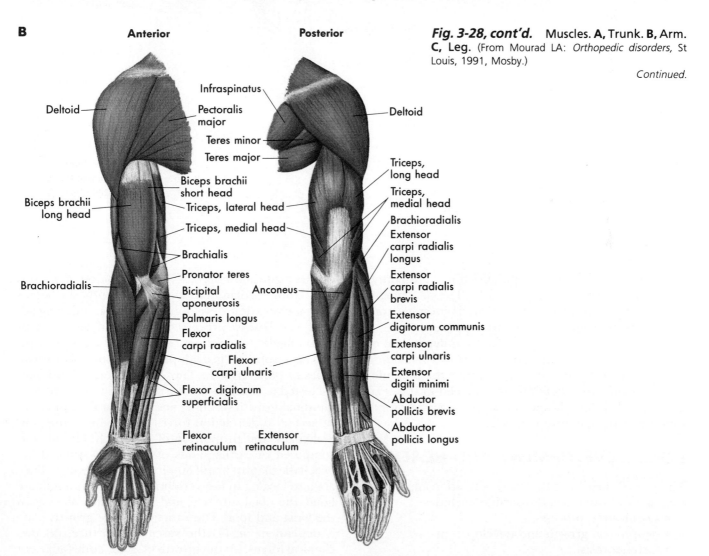

Fig. 3-28, cont'd.   Muscles. **A,** Trunk. **B,** Arm. **C, Leg.** (From Mourad LA: *Orthopedic disorders,* St Louis, 1991, Mosby.)

Continued.

Fig. 3-28, cont'd. Muscles. **A,** Trunk. **B,** Arm. **C,** Leg. (From Mourad LA: *Orthopedic disorders,* St Louis, 1991, Mosby.)

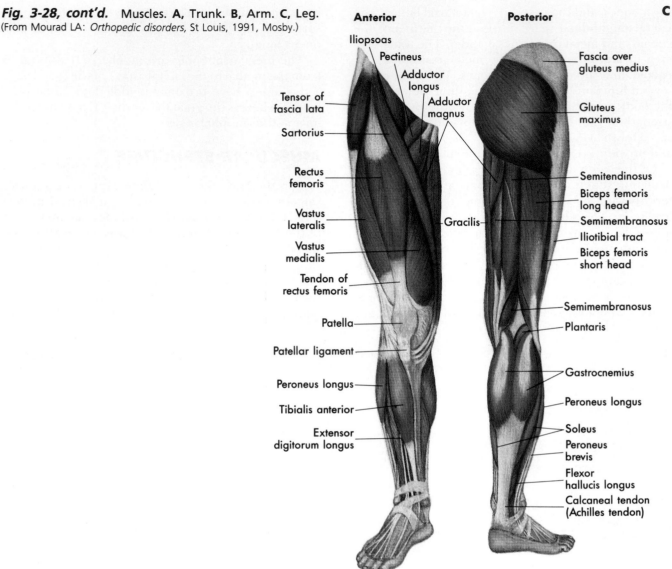

Anterior
- Iliopsoas
- Pectineus
- Adductor longus
- Tensor of fascia lata
- Adductor magnus
- Sartorius
- Rectus femoris
- Vastus lateralis
- Gracilis
- Vastus medialis
- Tendon of rectus femoris
- Patella
- Patellar ligament
- Peroneus longus
- Tibialis anterior
- Extensor digitorum longus

Posterior **C**
- Fascia over gluteus medius
- Gluteus maximus
- Semitendinosus
- Biceps femoris long head
- Semimembranosus
- Iliotibial tract
- Biceps femoris short head
- Semimembranosus
- Plantaris
- Gastrocnemius
- Peroneus longus
- Soleus
- Peroneus brevis
- Flexor hallucis longus
- Calcaneal tendon (Achilles tendon)

connective tissue covering; parallel fibers are bound together to form the entire muscle. The attachment of a muscle to bone or other tissue is indirect, connective tissue being used for this purpose.

The musculoskeletal system is not independent of other systems. There are other structures, including the neurovascular system, that support the musculoskeletal structure. These are not detailed in this text, although their significance must be noted in preparation for the operative procedure.

BONE DEVELOPMENT AND HEALING

The growth processes that have a relationship in the treatment of disease and disorders include:
- Ossification process
- Epiphyseal growth and development
- Osteoporosis

The ossification process is the formation of osseous cells from cartilaginous tissue. The process begins during embryonic development and ceases during adolescence. Disease processes, injury, and developmental anomalies may influence the ossification process.

The epiphyseal growth plate is responsible for two types of bone growth. Those plates located in bones subjected to compression forces contribute to the longitudinal growth of bone, and those located in bones subjected to distraction forces contribute to the general shape and proportion of the bone. The plate is composed of cartilaginous tissue and is situated between the diaphysis and epiphyses in long bones. They are also located in the vertebral bone, the innominate bone, the tibial tubercle, and small bones, such as in the wrist and foot. The function of the growth plate is dependent on (1) the vascular structure, (2) mechanical forces, (3) the growth of other bones adjacent to the plate, and (4) the presence or absence of abnormal physiologic factors.

Osteoporosis, a normal physiologic function that presents during adult (particularly older adult) years, results in increased porosity of the bone structure and cells due to gradual degeneration and resorption of cells. The process can be slowed or stopped by maintaining an active lifestyle and appropriate dietary habits. It is believed that the process is related to immobility and atrophy of musculature surrounding bone.

Bone healing begins when the integrity of the bone is damaged. The initial phase is localized inflammation. The bone end bleeds, and blood infiltrates the surrounding area, forming a hematoma. Fibroblasts invade the hematoma and form a fibrin network. Granulation tissue then replaces the hematoma. The second phase, cellular proliferation, includes invasion of the fibrin network by osteoblasts to develop collagen. Calcium deposits form in the granulation tissue to form a callus across the fracture site. The fracture is considered united at this stage.

The final stage of healing occurs when the primary cancellous bone is remodeled by new connective tissue cells. Compact bone is formed to strengthen the integrity of the site.

BIBLIOGRAPHY

Anthony CP, Thibodeau GA: *Textbook of anatomy and physiology*, ed 12, St Louis, 1987, Mosby.

Doyle JR: Anatomy of the finger flexor tendon sheath and pulley system, *J Hand Surg* 13:473, 1988.

Hansell MJ: Fractures and the healing process, *Orthop Nurs* 7:43, Jan/Feb 1988.

Hilt NE, Cogburn SB: *Manual of orthopedics*, St Louis, 1980, Mosby.

Meeker M, Rothrock J: *Alexander's care of the patient in surgery*, ed 9, St Louis, 1991, Mosby.

Mourad LA: *Orthopedic disorders*, St Louis, 1991, Mosby.

Reckling FW, Reckling JB, Mohn MP: *Orthopaedic anatomy and surgical approaches*, St Louis, 1990, Mosby.

Thibodeau GA, Patton KT: *Anatomy and physiology*, ed 2, St Louis, 1993, Mosby.

4

Perioperative Nursing Care

"Standards are authoritative statements by which the nursing profession describes the responsibilities for which its practitioners are accountable" (American Nurses Association, 1991). Written standards serve as a guideline providing direction for professional practice and a framework for evaluation of perioperative care. They provide a mechanism to judge the competency of nursing care that is provided by use of the nursing process, involving assessment, diagnosis, outcome identification, planning, implementation, and evaluation. The orthopaedic surgical patient is unique because of the procedure types and the other variables that must be considered for individualized care. The patient population crosses ranges of age, gender, and socioeconomic status, as well as cultural, racial, and ethnic diversity. Procedures are scheduled in an inpatient or an outpatient setting. Individuals differ in anatomic structure, as well as physiologic, psychologic, safety, functional, behavioral, knowledge, and home maintenance needs. Addressing these medical, surgical, anesthesia, and nursing needs is facilitated when those caring for the patient have a thorough understanding of orthopaedics as a specialty to individualize care.

Linking the nursing process to perioperative care is a necessary skill to avoid approaching patient care with a solely technical focus. Perioperative nurses are expected to assess, diagnose, plan, intervene, and evaluate rapidly, using time management and communication skills to accomplish this goal (see box). In most circumstances a perioperative nurse is dependent on the data and resources available at the time of the scheduled procedure. The essence of the role of a specialist involves independent judgment and activity initiated by the nurse.

CARE FOR SPECIAL POPULATIONS

The nursing process provides a systematic manner of providing care for different patient populations. Children and older adults commonly undergo orthopaedic procedures; because of their ages they have special needs. Effective care of pediatric populations must be tailored to individual children because their reactions are different from those of adults. Children's stress may be magnified by their parents' tension and anxiety, which can decrease the children's coping abilities. Parents or guardians of children undergoing ortho-

---

Standards of perioperative nursing clinical practice

I. Assessment: The perioperative nurse collects patient health data.

II. Diagnosis: The perioperative nurse analyzes the assessment data in determining diagnoses.

III. Outcome identification: The perioperative nurse identifies expected outcomes unique to the patient.

IV. Planning: The perioperative nurse develops a plan of care that prescribes interventions to attain expected outcomes.

V. Implementation: The perioperative nurse implements the interventions identified in the plan of care.

VI. Evaluation: The perioperative nurse evaluates the patient's progress toward attainment of expected outcomes.

From Association of Operating Room Nurses: *AORN standards and recommended practices*, Denver, 1993, AORN.

paedic procedures are resources for information needed to complete the assessment. Parental biases and needs must also be determined. During the assessment it is important to ensure that questions and comments are nonjudgmental, to prevent misinterpretation of the reason for the questions. Assessing perceptions of the surgical outcome to determine specific teaching and learning needs is valuable because parents often serve as the coach in the rehabilitation process. Intraoperative plans must be altered for children because of their poor thermoregulation and smaller fluid volume. Children, however, usually heal and recover rapidly.

As our population ages, the orthopaedic procedures required for the older age group also present opportunities and problems. The care of the older adult must take place in the context of an understanding of the normal aging process. The patient may be faced with dealing with a disability that causes fear or anxiety arising from an anticipated change in lifestyle, lack of understanding or knowledge, or a response to previous procedures. The older adult usually has adopted coping mechanisms to deal with some changes, but the nurse completing the assessment should determine whether these are appropriate or whether further assistance is needed. Older adults should specifically be assessed for the ability to resume activities early so as to reduce complications such as venous thrombosis or pulmonary embolism. Conditions common in the older adult, such as decreased vision and hearing, memory loss, and depression, may necessitate special considerations for communication. Relevant physiologic changes are summarized (see box).

Any individual, particularly a child or an older adult, is potentially a victim of abuse that may appear as an orthopaedic injury. The numbers of abused children and elderly persons are only estimates because of the lack of national registries for data gathering. Abuse is also inconsistently defined, resulting in questions arising as to the need to report it when the injury is identified. Abuse is generally described as intentional assault that produces injury, which could be physical or emotional in nature. It is estimated that over 1% of the pediatric population (Touloukian, 1990) and 2% to 4% of elderly persons are victims of abuse and neglect (AMA, Council on Scientific Affairs, 1987; Ferraro, 1990). Nurses often are the first persons to gather information that may result in discovery of injuries or behaviors requiring further investigation. It is important to approach the perioperative assessment with an awareness of the nurse's ability to play a critical role in patient care delivery in a scope broader than the intraoperative setting.

Changes in the older person's system

Integumentary
Decreased dermal thickness
Extended healing time
Decreased vascular responsiveness
Poor thermoregulation

Musculoskeletal
Decreased bone mass
Osteoarthrosis
Decreased intervertebral disk space
Calcification of joint margins
Decreased muscle mass
Impaired motor function and strength

Respiratory
Decreased ciliary action
Less effective gas exchange
Decreased vital capacity

Cardiovascular
Less effective cardiac output
Delayed stress response
Arterial stiffness, leading to hypertension
Increased left ventricular workload

Sensory Functioning
Reduced visual acuity
Presbyopia

From Booth B, Kumar A: Surgery for elderly patients: a new specialty? *Nurs Times* 85:26, July 1989.

COMMUNICATION

Skillful communication is a basic element of the nursing process, particularly in the perioperative environment, where the amount of time for communication with the patient and family is minimal. Verbal and nonverbal communication skills should be developed to gather information for the purpose of planning patient care. Communication with patients is enhanced in a comfortable environment. Noise and lack of privacy or space may create tension, discomfort, and confusion. The perioperative nurse has the responsibility to eliminate as many environmental distractions as possible to enhance communication. Communication techniques must be adjusted to meet the needs of the individual if there are barriers. Physically active individuals requiring surgery may feel threatened by their questionable return to activity. Older patients may be experiencing those same feelings for different reasons. Both groups of patients require an intense psychosocial assessment, including nursing intervention to modify the environment to match the patient's needs and to determine the best time for an assessment, if possible.

In addition to patient communication, many other disciplines are involved in planning the operative procedure. The timing, data gathering, and method of communication with others can decrease the potential for delays and the stress on perioperative team members and improve patient care.

ASSESSMENT

Collection of client health data provides information for an effective nursing assessment that will identify patterns of deviation to use in the remaining phases of the nursing process. The goal of the preoperative assessment is data collection for identification of nursing diagnosis, communication of information, and continuation of the nursing process. The perioperative nurse is responsible for completing a thorough assessment to begin the planning phase of the perioperative experience. Varying degrees of assessments will have been performed on surgical patients before admission. The typically healthy patient may have had only a physical examination for the orthopaedic problem being treated, with minimal review of other systems. A patient with previous medical problems may have had an intensive medical assessment but only minimal psychologic assessment. Perioperative nurses should always conduct their own physical and psychologic assessment on the patient's admission to provide accurate measures of health and function.

The perioperative nurse completes an assessment of the patient undergoing orthopaedic procedures in a variety of settings. Assessments are completed in the physician's office, surgical inpatient unit, preoperative holding, or other areas depending on the organization of the setting. An attempt should be made to complete the assessment before the patient arrives for the surgical procedure. Many individuals interact with the patient during the initial preoperative phase, including a nurse or physician's assistant who works in the physician's office. For continuity, it is valuable for the nurse caring for the patient during the procedure to maintain contact with personnel initially involved in the assessment phase.

The variety of orthopaedic procedures completed requires utilization of skills to synthesize information and individualize patient care appropriate for the procedure being planned. An accurate assessment of the patient before his or her arrival in the surgical suite can significantly decrease confusion and intraoperative time. This should be considered a priority for the care of every patient. General information that should

be ascertained in the assessment of every patient undergoing a surgical procedure includes:

- Verification of the patient and the operative site
- Correct, complete consent for the procedure and blood administration as applicable
- Understanding of the anesthetic to be administered

Assessment information specific to care of the orthopaedic patient may include medical status; previous surgical procedures; the presence of implants, prostheses, or external fixation devices; physical condition; psychologic status; preoperative preparation; and results of tests or diagnostic procedures. These are each discussed in the following sections.

Medical Status

The medical status review should include cardiac, respiratory, renal, and neurovascular status; cause(s) of medical needs; nutritional status; medication history; allergies to medications, foods, or chemicals; skin conditions; and sensory impairments. Assessment of the medical status of the patient, including the history and impairments or other problems that have been diagnosed and/or treated, should be completed by the perioperative nurse. Medical conditions can increase the surgical risk to patients undergoing orthopaedic procedures. Patients who appear healthy should always be assessed for potential medical conditions that may affect the plan of care. Medical conditions that increase the surgical risk include bleeding disorders, diabetes mellitus, heart disease, infection, fever, and chronic respiratory disease. Nutritional status should be evaluated to determine positioning and postoperative protection needs. The medication history of the patient with orthopaedic disorders is important to determine because over-the-counter medications may increase the risk of hemorrhaging or cause adverse effects of anesthesia. Noted allergies determine the appropriateness of routine skin preparation solutions and medications administered. Skin conditions such as a rash or abrasions may prohibit the surgical procedure because of the possibility of increasing the chances of postoperative infection. Medical conditions can require attention during the procedure or the postoperative phase and should be considered as important as the orthopaedic condition being treated.

Previous Surgical Procedures

Previous surgical procedures, including the type of procedure, patient's response to the procedure physically and emotionally, patient's response to the anesthetic, patient's postoperative recovery, and patient's significant memories of the surgical experience, should be assessed. Patients undergoing surgical intervention are influenced by past experiences to prepare them for the surgical procedure. Understanding their perceptions and recollections assists the nurse in developing the plan of care to include actions that will provide support for the patient. The nurse should explore personal recollections of surgical experiences, as well as information shared by friends and family. Assessment should also include postoperative experiences related to the previous surgery.

Presence of Implantable Devices

Assessment for the presence of implantable devices, including the type and location of prostheses, plates, screws, wires, and external fixators, is important before any procedures are completed to plan nursing activities. This information assists in planning safety needs such as transfer, positioning, and placement of an electrosurgical pad. Restricted range of motion caused by presence of a fixator assists in planning positioning and padding needs. Instruments needed for removing or replacing an implant must be anticipated for the implementation phase of the procedure.

Physical Condition

The patient's physical condition, including congenital or acquired impairments, range of motion, muscle and skin integrity, height and weight, and nutritional status, is part of assessment. Patients with altered physical conditions require attention during the intraoperative phase to ensure a safe outcome. The cause of alteration may be medical conditions or previous procedures. Examples include the presence of scar tissue, a limited range of motion, excess body mass, the absence of extremities, or paralysis. Nutritional status may impact the opportunity for postoperative infection (Smith, 1991), requiring a high level of awareness of intraoperative techniques. These considerations of the patient's physical conditions are important for intraoperative planning related to the method of patient transfer and positioning, placement of the electrosurgical unit ground pad, or other needs. They may also impede postoperative recovery and require assessment to determine the patient's teaching and learning needs.

Psychologic Status

Patients undergoing an elective orthopaedic procedure as their first surgical experience, as well as individuals who have undergone several surgical procedures, must be assessed for their response to the anticipated procedure. The outcome of the procedure may depend on their willingness to participate and their understanding of the rehabilitation process. Patients must be prepared for the pain they may experience postoperatively, and they must learn about

the mechanisms of controlling pain, as well as their role in the surgical outcome. Assessing the family's response is beneficial in determining the available support system. The patient's ability to understand teaching or instructions must be assessed. Meeting an individual's level of comprehension can influence that person's anxiety level and postoperative response.

Preoperative Preparation

Preoperative preparation varies according to the surgeon's preferences and the surgical procedure planned. All patients, particularly outpatients, must be assessed for intake status to avoid intraoperative complications. Patients may be required to begin antibiotics 2 to 3 days before the procedure. They may also be instructed to clean the operative site with an antibacterial solution. Orthopaedic procedures often require shaving of the surgical site immediately before the procedure. The site should be assessed for abrasions, cuts, or a rash. Assessment by the nurse requires an understanding of the physician's preferences and the ability to accurately determine compliance with instructions.

Tests and Diagnostic Procedures

Tests and procedures required before orthopaedic procedures are done vary. The perioperative nurse must be familiar with tests routinely completed for procedures, such as blood tests, electrocardiograms, and chest x-ray films, in addition to special tests for orthopaedic procedures. Valuable information can be gained from reviewing the results of these tests before the patient is brought to surgery. Laboratory values and other test results may indicate an insidious infection, need for blood availability, or an undetected arrhythmia. It is important to recognize subtle changes in test results that can indicate a medical problem requiring attention. Many non-trauma-related orthopaedic procedures can be scheduled to allow treatment and correction of a medical problem before the surgical procedure is done.

Diagnostic procedures for musculoskeletal diseases and disorders are completed to determine the need or extent of surgery required. Most are completed before the need for surgery is determined, but some may be completed in the operating room. The results of diagnostic procedures must be available before the procedure is done. These procedures supplement an accurate history, clinical examination, and an understanding of the relationship to normal anatomic findings.

Invasive diagnostic procedures

Arthrography is the introduction of air or radiopaque dye (or sometimes both for a double-contrast arthrography) into a joint cavity to facilitate visualization of joint structures, including ligaments, tendons, and cartilage. An arthrography can be performed on any joint but usually is used to diagnose symptoms of the knee and shoulder. The use of arthroscopy has decreased the need for knee studies. Shoulder arthrography has its greatest application in the study of rotator cuff tears. Excess joint fluid is aspirated, and air or dye is injected. The joint is manipulated, and multiple films are taken during the procedure.

Bone marrow aspiration or biopsy permits microscopic examination of bone marrow obtained through closed (needle aspiration) or open means. A needle biopsy can be accomplished by fine-needle aspiration or core biopsy. A bone biopsy is frequently required for investigation of systemic skeletal disorders, such as osteoporosis, osteomalacia, hyperparathyroidism, and renal osteodystrophy. A biopsy specimen can be taken from one or more sites for the purpose of systemic diagnosis. A bone biopsy is also required for diagnosis of localized skeletal pathologic conditions.

Intraoperatively a Craig biopsy needle may be requested for aspiration if an open biopsy procedure is not deemed necessary. A tissue biopsy can be done through an incision with removal of enough tissue for histologic examination. The tissue can be bone or muscle.

Joint aspiration is withdrawal of synovial fluid for joint aspiration by inserting a needle into the synovial capsule of the joint for microscopic examination. This procedure may also be performed for pain relief when effusion and joint swelling are evident.

Noninvasive diagnostic procedures

Bone scintigraphy is a procedure for detecting bone metastasis or stress fracture. It may be necessary if the metastasis cannot be detected with radiographic examination. Primary tumors can be diagnosed 3 to 6 months earlier than their detection with radiographic examination. A bone scan is not useful in detecting soft tissue malignancy.

Computed tomography (CT) is reliable for confirming a suspected bone, joint, or soft tissue abnormality. It describes the marrow and soft tissue extent in the transverse plane and the relationship to nerves and vessels. The accuracy of CT scans depends on the presence of fat in the surrounding soft tissues to define individual muscles, vessels, and nerves. The CT scan includes a series of 8-mm to 1-cm sections from one end of the suspected pathologic area to the other, including normal regions.

Electromyography (EMG) is a method of determining the electrical potential generated in an individual muscle. The electrical activity generated

through the insertion of a sterile needle electrode into the specific muscle is amplified and displayed on a cathode ray oscilloscope. The diagnosis of muscle denervation, level or area of nerve injury, presence of dystrophies and myopathies, or recurrence of innervation can be accomplished.

Laboratory tests on blood and other fluids can provide a diagnosis or confirmation of the diagnosis. Understanding laboratory values can also determine musculoskeletal implications.

Abnormal fluids collected from the area of bone, soft tissue, or bursa in the musculoskeletal system are examined grossly, microscopically, and using blood chemistry procedures. The results vary for the type of specimen collected.

Blood specimens are collected routinely on every patient. The results of the blood specimen studies may indicate an orthopaedic problem or other medical conditions requiring attention before a surgical procedure is initiated. The complete blood count (CBC), including hemoglobin, hematocrit, red blood cell count, white blood cell count, and microscopic examination, aids in diagnosing infection, arthritis, and some tumors. Other diagnostic studies will be ordered for assessment of a musculoskeletal disorder (see Table 4-1).

Magnetic resonance imaging (MRI) is a technique using magnetic and radiofrequency fields to produce images of the internal structures of the body. It does not involve ionizing radiation and is capable of imaging in multiple planes (sagittal, coronal, transverse, and oblique). It can provide superior soft tissue contrast of muscle, ligament, tendon, fat, and fluid, giving a more complete view of pathologic changes to assist in diagnosis. The technique involves placing a patient in a strong magnetic field and stimulating the anatomic hydrogen nuclei (protons) with a radio transmission. The available tissue contrast is the highest among all medical imaging modalities. Most patients are a candidate for this examination, since there are few untoward effects or contraindications known. A patient who is not in stable condition usually cannot undergo MRI, since close monitoring cannot be accomplished in the scanner. Conscious patients in severe pain may not be able to undergo this procedure because of motion artifacts.

A **myelogram** provides visualization of lesions or defects of the spinal column by introduction of a radiopaque dye into the subarachnoid space. The myelogram can be used to diagnose herniated intervertebral disks, spinal cord compression, tumors, vascular anomalies, and bone structure defects.

Radiography is an x-ray examination used for diagnosis of orthopaedic conditions preoperatively. Intraoperatively it is used to verify the location or align-

Table 4-1 ■ *Diagnostic studies used for assessment of the musculoskeletal system*

Laboratory study	Orthopaedic relevance	Normal value
Acid phosphatase	Elevated in multiple myeloma, carcinoma of bone (primary and metastatic)	0.10-0.63 U/ml (Bessey-Lowry); 0.5-2.0 U/ml (Bodansky); 1.0-4.0 U/ml (King-Armstrong)
Alkaline phosphatase	Elevated in healing fractures, rheumatoid arthritis, osteogenic sarcoma, osteomalacia	30-85 (lmU/ml)
Antinuclear antibody test (ANA)	Elevated (positive titer) in systemic lupus erythematosus (SLE), rheumatoid arthritis	Absence of antinuclear bodies detected at 1 : 32 titer
Creatinine phosphokinase (CPK)	Elevated in insult to skeletal muscle	5-75 mU/ml
C-Reactive protein (CRP)	Elevated in rheumatoid arthritis, malignancies	<60 U/ml
Erythrocyte sedimentation rate (ESR)	Elevated with bone, cartilage, soft tissue destruction, osteomyelitis, gout	Males: 0-20 mm/hr Females: 0-30 mm/hr (Westergren)
Lactic dehydrogenase (LDH)	Elevated with muscle tissue damage, malignancy	90-200 lmU/ml
LE cell prep	Elevated in SLE	Absence of LE cells
Phosphorus (serum)	Elevated in osteoporosis, bone fracture healing; lowered with hypercalcemia, osteomalacia	1.8-2.6 mEq/L or 3-4.5 mg/dl
Rheumatoid factor test	Elevated (positive titer) in rheumatoid arthritis	Absence of rheumatoid factor
Serum asparate aminotransferase (AST; formerly SGOT)	Elevated in primary muscle disease, crush injuries	5-40 IU/L
Serum calcium	Elevated (hypercalcemia) in metastatic tumor to bone; elevated or depressed in metabolic disease	9.0-10.5 mg/dl (total)
Uric acid (serum)	Elevated (hyperuricemia) in gout, arthritis, soft tissue deposits of uric acid (tophi), low-dose aspirin therapy	Male: 2.1-8.5 mg/dl Female: 2.0-6.6 mg/dl

Modified from Rothrock JC: *Perioperative nursing care planning,* St Louis, 1990, Mosby.

ment of a structure. Radiation is transmitted in the form of a beam to visualize bone structure and function. X-ray films show density changes, irregularities in contour, changes in the shape of a bone or joint, and the presence of soft tissue swelling. Bony areas may be visualized, but details needed for comparison of soft tissue masses with dense tissue and bone may not be visible. Two views of the bone at right angles is taken for diagnostic interpretation.

Venography is visualization of the venous system in the lower extremity. Radiographic diagnosis is used to determine the presence or absence of thrombosis and general venous competence. Upper extremity venography may be accomplished, although it is rarely indicated. Radiopaque dye is injected in an area distal to the defect and allowed to flow proximally.

DIAGNOSIS

The perioperative nurse analyzes the assessment data in determining diagnoses. Individualized nursing diagnoses can be determined following the assessment, based on the medical history, previous surgical experiences, presence of implants or prostheses, physical condition, psychologic response, laboratory val-

ues, and diagnostic data. They should be validated with the client, significant others, and health care providers. Documentation of diagnoses facilitates determination of the expected outcomes and plan of care. Examples of nursing diagnoses from the accepted list developed by the North American Nursing Diagnosis Association (NANDA) that may be determined for the orthopaedic patient include the following:

Sensory/perceptual alterations
High risk for infection
High risk for impaired tissue integrity
Impaired physical mobility
Body image disturbance
Altered tissue perfusion
High risk for trauma
High risk for injury
Pain
High risk for altered body temperature
High risk for fluid volume deficit
High risk for impaired skin integrity
Altered nutrition: less than body requirements
Altered nutrition: more than body requirements
Knowledge deficit
Anxiety
Fear

OUTCOME IDENTIFICATION

The perioperative nurse identifies expected outcomes unique to the patient. Patient outcomes are derived from the nursing diagnoses and anticipated results of the plan of care, and are individualized for each diagnosis. Respect for the patient's goals and preferences should be a priority when there is a choice to promote involvement and independence. These may include:

- Absence of infection
- Skin integrity maintained
- Absence of adverse results of positioning; safety measures provided
- Maintenance of fluid and electrolyte balance
- Thermal regulation for patient comfort
- Understanding of the perioperative experience
- Fear and/or anxiety expressed and alleviated or managed
- Management of pain
- Participation in the rehabilitation process

Outcomes should be attainable, considering the resources available for the patient. They should also be able to be measured and communicated for ongoing intraoperative and postoperative evaluation.

PLANNING

The perioperative nurse develops a plan of care that prescribes interventions to attain expected outcomes. Patients' needs and goals are identified from information gathered during the assessment process. The plan should include:

- Ensuring development of a teaching plan, including provision of information specific to the orthopaedic procedure and intended outcome
- Verifying the surgical site and understanding the surgical procedure and expectations
- Ensuring availability of competent personnel, functional equipment, and appropriate supplies
- Determining transport needs
- Identifying the type of anesthetic to be administered
- Adhering to policies and procedures based on AORN Recommended Practices for Perioperative Nursing Care (Association of Operating Room Nurses, 1993) including infection control practices, safety practices, and documentation.

Planning patient care will improve the organization and efficiency of the orthopaedic nurse during the implementation of care. Planning begins at the time the procedure is posted and requires coordination among the surgeon, office staff, nurses, and anesthesia personnel responsible for care to meet the unique needs of each patient. The evolution of sophisticated and highly technical procedures has increased the responsibility of the nurse specializing in orthopaedics. Organizing the procedure by using a plan of care is an effective means of decreasing intraoperative time and providing safe patient care. A documented plan can also be used to determine methods for improved care through evaluation.

Patient Teaching

Patient teaching plans for an orthopaedic procedure are individualized following the preoperative assessment. Patient needs can be met if the teaching is planned with consideration for the specific psychologic, spiritual, and physical needs of each patient in relation to each procedure. Teaching should begin at the time the patient decides to have the surgical procedure done; the perioperative nurse's responsibility and length of time for teaching will vary in different environments. Teaching the following general information about the preoperative, intraoperative, and postoperative phases will prepare the patient for the procedure and postoperative expectations.

Preoperative phase
- Cause of injury or disease process
- Diagnostic tests
- Surgical procedure and expected outcome
- Anticipated routines before surgery
- Operating room environment

Intraoperative phase
- Preoperative area, operating room, and postanesthesia care environment
- Waiting areas for significant others or family; anticipated length of procedure
- Anticipated length of postanesthesia care unit (PACU) stay

Postoperative phase
- Symptoms of complications and expected response
- Rehabilitation process, including length, physical therapy, exercises, limitation of activities
- Use of assistive devices, including crutches, braces
- Care of external fixators, dressings

Unless a procedure is completed immediately following trauma, patients experiencing bone and joint disorders may have withstood preoperative discomfort or pain for long periods of time, causing them to seek surgical intervention. Although such patients realize the limitations caused by the disorder, they must be prepared for short and long-term postoperative management. Patients must realize that postoperative pain may be experienced, requiring medication for relief. They should be taught that pain is expected and that medication should be taken before the severity of the pain is intolerable or before physical therapy is started. The method of administration of pain medication will vary. Patients undergoing procedures as an outpatient generally receive pain medications with a low-dosage narcotic. Patients undergoing procedures as an inpatient, such as for total joint replacement, may receive pain medications with the patient-controlled analgesic (PCA) pump. The method of administration and patient cautions should be reinforced preoperatively and postoperatively.

Patients undergoing orthopaedic procedures may or may not have experienced previous surgical procedures. Patients sometimes undergo multiple orthopaedic procedures for one disorder. Their expectations will alter their response to patient teaching, nursing care, and even the outcome of the procedure. Orthopaedic nurses should continually assess and plan comfort measures and supportive care for patients and families.

Procedure Verification

Verification of the procedure should be part of the routine for orthopaedic procedures, since they are commonly performed on extremities or areas with bilateral anatomic structures, such as the lumbar spine. Verifying the correct patient and surgical site assists in planning for room preparation, equipment availability, and instrument needs. The information gathered from the patient should be compared with reports of diagnostic tests to ensure that planning is complete for the procedure. Patients should be able to verbalize their understanding of the procedure. Assessment of their understanding and willingness to discuss the procedure assists in planning teaching and supportive activities.

Personnel, Equipment, and Supplies

Personnel, equipment, and supply needs vary for each orthopaedic procedure that is scheduled. Room selection may be based on the operative site or amount of equipment needed for the procedure. Product representatives play a key role in the procedure by ensuring the availability of necessary supplies. A plan to ensure that stock supply is maintained must be a priority of personnel responsible for the orthopaedic specialty. Unsterile instruments and implants must be available for sterilization before the procedure to allow packaging and sterilization in a sterilizer load with a biologic monitor. Positioning aids or special equipment such as the fracture table or fluoroscopy must also be available.

Scheduling also requires ensuring the availability of personnel with the appropriate skill level to provide for patient safety and decrease anesthesia time and tissue exposure. Caring for orthopaedic patients is a physically strenuous responsibility. Assistants with experience are needed during transport of the patient to the operating room, positioning, patient preparations, performance of the procedure, and postoperative transfer. The orthopaedic staff includes personnel other than those in circulating and scrub roles to complete the team. Personnel assisting with transfer, positioning, and holding extremities should be educated to meet the specific needs of orthopaedic patients. Each institution handles this staffing need differently. Some orthopaedic surgeons employ registered nurses to function in the role of RN first assistant (RNFA), providing direct patient care in a specialized role.

Patient Transport

Transport of orthopaedic patients to the operating room is sometimes complicated by the status of an injury. Patients undergoing elective procedures may not have the difficulty in moving of those with traumatic injuries, who may be in traction or immobilizers. Complicated traumatic injuries are painful to the patient when moving, requiring an understanding by the transporter of the anatomic alignment or the need to obtain assistance. Personnel moving a bed with a patient in it should always have enough assistance to transport the patient without causing injury to the patient or themselves. Traction devices should be held to prevent swinging, and extremities or injured areas should be mobilized from movement.

Anesthetics

Anesthetic administration for orthopaedic patients is a specialized activity. Each type of anesthetic delivered requires an understanding by the perioperative nurse of the medication, the method of delivery, and any complications. Patients must also understand the procedures for the type of anesthetic to be delivered and the outcome expected. A patient scheduled for spinal anesthesia requires appropriate planning for transfer to the perioperative setting in adequate time to allow administration of the spinal. Patients undergoing procedures on the upper extremity may receive a Bier block, requiring emotional support for the patient and availability of supplies for the procedure.

Physiologic effects differ with the type of anesthetic chosen. Choice depends on a combination of factors, including patient preference, coexisting disease, anatomy, absence of contraindications, operative site, length of procedure, and position (see box on p. 37).

Regional anesthetics are given epidurally, spinally, by axillary block, by interscalene block, and by intravenous regional anesthesia. Epidural anesthesia may be given to a patient undergoing orthopaedic procedures both during the procedure and/or for postoperative pain. An epidural catheter is inserted before the operation or in the operating room. Epidural anesthesia is the injection of a local anesthetic solution

Comparison of anesthetics

General	Regional
Renders patient unconscious with need to protect airway	Sedative for sleep, but consciousness and airway maintained
Onset rapid	Onset within 5 to 30 minutes
High rate of success	Failure rate approximately 10%
Physiologic effects	Physiologic effects
Myocardial depression	Does not inhibit contractility or respiration
Inhibited respiration	
Muscle relaxation	Muscle relaxation causes regional sympathectomy
	Decreased intraoperative bleeding
Associated complications	Associated complications
Airway management	Local anesthetic toxicity
Cardiovascular effects	Hypotension

or narcotic into the epidural space. When a continuous infusion is given, supplemental anesthetic can be injected periodically through a catheter threaded into the epidural space.

Spinal anesthesia (subarachnoid block) has a higher success rate (greater than 95%) than epidural anesthesia. The anesthetic is injected in the subarachnoid space. Unless a catheter is placed for repeat injection, the anesthetic has a finite duration. Spinal anesthesia reduces blood loss, decreases thromboembolitic complications, and preserves mental acuity in the older adult. A complication of spinal anesthesia is postoperative headache.

An axillary block is accomplished by perivascular infiltration of a local anesthetic into the axillary sheath. It is used to block the distal brachial plexus for sensory and motor innervation of the hand, wrist, forearm, and elbow. It is successful in 90% to 95% of cases. Problems that can occur include tourniquet pain and neuropathies. This block is not always reliable in shoulder and elbow procedures.

The interscalene block is a regional block for the proximal brachial plexus. Advantages over the axillary block are anesthetization of both the shoulder and the upper arm and the ability to perform the block in any position.

Intravenous regional anesthesia was described in 1908 by Bier, resulting in the Bier block technique that bears his name. A double tourniquet is applied proximally to the operative site. After limb exsanguination, the tourniquet is inflated, and local anesthetic (0.5%) without epinephrine is then slowly injected intravenously. It is an effective method for obtaining rapid analgesia of the forearm and hand, used during procedures less than 1 hour in length. It can be effective for 60 to 90 minutes, but patients will complain of tourniquet pain within 60 minutes. The double cuff provides 30 to 40 more minutes of analgesia. This type of analgesia is not recommended for lower extremity procedures because of the large volume of anesthetic needed when the tourniquet is placed on the thigh. If the tourniquet is placed over the calf, it is difficult to obtain and maintain adequate exsanguination (Gravenstein, 1991).

Intraoperative Planning

An intraoperative plan is an effective means of decreasing surgical time, providing safe patient care, and determining methods for improving care. The simplest procedure can become complex without appropriate planning by the perioperative nurse.

Policies and procedures are written as guidelines for implementing care and must be considered when planning care. The Association of Operating Room Nurses has written recommended practices applicable to the intraoperative setting that should be used as a basis for determining policies and procedures. These recommended practices provide guidelines for care of patients undergoing surgical procedures and should be adapted to meet the needs of orthopaedic patients. The activities to be implemented require planning for organization of personnel, traffic control, and patient protection during the procedure. Policies and procedures should include infection control practices such as aseptic techniques and traffic patterns, safety practices for equipment use and patient care, and documentation.

Aseptic practices and traffic patterns are established to decrease the opportunity for infections. Activities should be planned to control and minimize movement of personnel and traffic flow through the room in a pattern that eliminates movement around the sterile field. Bacteria counts increase as air travels through the operating room. Shedding of contaminated particles from the patient, personnel, and drapes increases with movement throughout the room. Prioritizing activities and equipment placement in the room will facilitate traffic flow and progression of the procedure. Time should be allowed to check equipment for function before moving the patient to the room. The room should be selected to allow the patient to be positioned where traffic flow can be prevented near the sterile field. Equipment and supplies should be placed to minimize traffic near the surgical site and maximize visibility by the scrubbed personnel.

Physician preferences play a key role in planning and implementing patient care. Physicians must have confidence in the operating room personnel. This can be achieved by ensuring that the team understands the procedure and the rationale for the physician's preferences, recognizes the patient's needs, and plans activities to improve the outcome. Preoperative planning should be shared with all team members, including the physician, to benefit the patient.

IMPLEMENTATION

The perioperative nurse implements the interventions identified in the plan of care. Surgical interventions should be consistent with the plan of care that has been individualized to meet the patient's needs and then documented. Each step of the plan is implemented, evaluated, and adjusted for appropriateness during patient care. The procedures identified in this book are a guide for implementation by personnel caring for the patient. The responsibilities for implementation will vary depending on the procedure being completed, the physician's preferences, and the roles of personnel. The registered nurse is responsible for implementing the plan of care. Activities to be implemented include patient teaching, assurance of safety, positioning, documentation, and infection control measures.

Patient Teaching

Patient teaching needs are continual, requiring assessment, planning, implementation, and evaluation from the time the patient initially visits the physician to the end of the rehabilitation process. Several individuals may be responsible for patient teaching. Collaboration among those responsible will enhance the perioperative experience for the patient. The perioperative nurse can provide a supportive environment for the patient and family, considering their special needs. This can be accomplished by developing a teaching program (Orr, 1990) to provide both information and emotional support. Immediately before

surgery, previous instructions, such as those regarding postoperative complications, rehabilitation, and expectations, can be reinforced. A physical therapist may be available to teach crutch walking, special exercises, or other therapy. Nursing personnel may review pin site care, cast care, or medication therapy. Individuals undergoing procedures as outpatients or those with special learning needs will benefit from repetition and preoperative and postoperative return demonstrations.

Safety

Safety measures for the patient and personnel during implementation of the plan are necessary during orthopaedic procedures. Safety during patient transport, transfer, and positioning requires adequate numbers of personnel familiar with the appropriate techniques and responsibilities. Equipment safety measures and environmental hazards should be addressed during the orientation and education of personnel caring for orthopaedic patients because of the equipment used and necessary environmental precautions. Personnel should be familiar with chemicals present in the setting, including skin preparation solutions, glutaraldehydes, and methylmethacrylate, and hazards of improper use.

Positioning

Positioning orthopaedic patients requires an understanding of the basic positions and variations required for procedures to meet patient needs in addition to physician preferences, available equipment, and proper use. The success of some orthopaedic procedures may depend on the surgical position; therefore the time spent positioning and assessing the outcome is important.

Common positions for orthopaedic procedures are dorsal recumbent (supine), prone, and lateral decubitus. Patient positions are modified using special equipment to accommodate the desired anatomic approach, the technique required for the procedure, and the physical limitations of the patient. Physicians commonly have a preference if specialized equipment is required for positioning. Positions are identified for each procedure shown.

Orthopaedic surgeons maintain an active role in positioning because of the physical requirements and the need to protect the involved anatomic structure. Priority positioning considerations are unrestricted thoracic movement, protected neuromuscular and skin integrity, and maintained body alignment.

Intervention is determined by preoperative assessment of positioning needs. Assessment should include physical limitations, height and weight, type and length of the procedure, nutritional status, skin con-

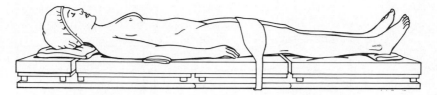

Fig. 4-1 Dorsal recumbent (supine) position.

dition, and preexisting disease to ensure appropriate-size positioning devices and adequate numbers of personnel.

Padding extremities, bony prominences, and compromised areas should be considered for every patient, even when procedures do not take much time (Vermillion, 1990). Padding on operating room beds may be sufficient for patient protection if the patient has adequate skin and neuromuscular integrity. Because of the unusual positions sometimes required for orthopaedic procedures, prevention of peripheral nerve injury must be considered a priority. If the extremity or body part is near the edge of the bed or a positioning device, movement during the procedure can result in unnecessary nerve or tissue damage if the body part is not protected.

Dorsal recumbent (supine) position

This position permits access to anterior surfaces of the body (Fig. 4-1). The patient is placed on his or her back with arms extended parallel to the body or angled at the sides. The head, vertebrae, hips, and legs should be in alignment. A small pad placed beneath the head prevents neck strain. The legs should be slightly separated to prevent peroneal and tibial nerve damage, compromised circulation, and skin breakdown. A restraint is placed across the mid- to upper thighs, loosely enough to prevent circulatory compromise. A procedure on one lower extremity may require placing the restraining strap across only the remaining extremity. The arms resting at the side of the body should have the palms against the body or pronated (palm down) on the mattress and secured. Arms placed on the armboard should be at less than a 90-degree angle to the body with palms up. The mattress and armboard pad should be the same height with the same amount of padding to prevent nerve damage.

The dorsal recumbent (supine) position is modified for procedures requiring access to the surgical site. These include procedures on the shoulder or the knee and procedures requiring positioning on the fracture table. Positioning principles apply to modified positions with consideration of the pressure points and areas to be protected. A patient may be positioned for

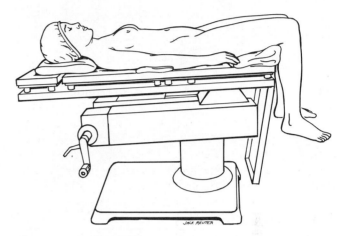

Fig. 4-2 Modified supine position for arthroscopic knee procedures.

knee procedures (arthroscopy, meniscectomy, anterior cruciate ligament repair) in a modified supine position (Fig. 4-2). The patient is placed on the operating room bed with the knees at the "break" in the table, where the lower portion of the table is hinged. Following induction, the foot section of the table is lowered to 90 degrees. A knee holder may be used to secure the knee requiring the procedure, with the safety strap secured across the opposite thigh. The position affords distraction of the tibial plateaus from the femoral condyles, increasing the width of the joint space. Pressure on the popliteal fossa must be avoided. A modified supine position is used for shoulder procedures, with the bed slightly flexed and the patient positioned so that the affected shoulder is near the edge of the bed (Fig. 4-3). Protection of vulnerable areas is similar to that for the supine position.

Lateral decubitus position

Access to anatomic sites on the side of the patient can be accomplished with the patient in this position (Fig. 4-4). Modified lateral positions may also be used for procedures on the hip and shoulder. The patient is anesthetized in the supine position and turned to the unaffected side. The position is described as right or left lateral, identifying the side on which the patient is lying. A minimum of four persons is required for

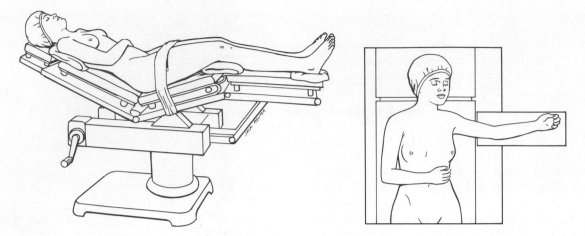

Fig. 4-3   Modified supine position for shoulder procedures.

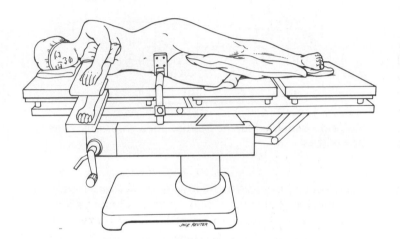

Fig. 4-4   Lateral position.

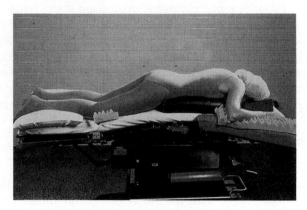

Fig. 4-5   Prone position on chest rolls.

lateral positioning. Positioning devices, such as braces, a three-point positioner, or a surgical positioning system (Vacpac), are used to stabilize the torso throughout the procedure. The torso is secured. With the patient in a full lateral decubitus position, an axillary roll is placed to protect the neurovascular structures and shoulder joints. The legs are positioned by flexing the bottom leg at the hip and knee. The top leg is frequently draped free and manipulated during the procedure. A restraining strap may be used if necessary. Pressure points to be assessed include the ear, the acromion process, the iliac crest, the greater trochanter, the medial and lateral knee, and the malleolus.

Prone position

The prone position (Fig. 4-5) is used for access to the posterior surfaces of the body. The patient is anesthetized in the supine position on the transport stretcher or bed. Following intubation and after en-

suring that the endotrachial tube is secured, the patient is turned onto the abdomen. Before the patient is turned, pedal pulses should be evaluated for presence and strength. Positioning devices, such as chest bolsters or other equipment, are placed lengthwise from the acromioclavicular joint to the iliac crests to elevate the chest, permitting the diaphragm to move freely and lung expansion to occur.

Moving the patient into position and ensuring correct positioning requires at least four persons. The anesthesiologist supports the head and neck and ensures that respiration is maintained during and following the move. One person assumes responsibility for initiating the "logroll" by placing his or her hands at the shoulder and buttock of the patient and gently turning the patient onto the arms of the second person on the opposite side. One person supports and turns the legs during positioning. Following the turn, correct positioning of the body and arms must be ensured. The arms are positioned on armboards at each

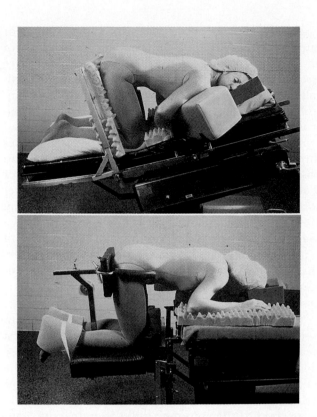

Fig. 4-6 Two modifications of knee-chest position using positioning frames.

side of the bed. The arms are moved through normal range of motion by bringing them down and forward to rest on the armboards with the elbows flexed and hands pronated. Areas to be assessed for protective padding include the eyes, ears, breasts of females, iliac crests, genitalia of males, knees, and toes. Following positioning, the pedal pulses should be checked for presence and strength. Absence of a pedal pulse may require evaluation and repositioning of the positioning device on the affected side.

A modified knee-chest position (Fig. 4-6) can be used for procedures on the lower vertebrae using positioning devices or beds designed for this purpose. Positioning requires a minimum of four persons for the safety of the patient and personnel. The patient is initially positioned prone. Two persons assume responsibility for lifting the chest of the patient, and bolsters are placed beneath the chest as the bed is moved into Trendelenburg's position. The buttocks rest on a frame placed on the bed. The arms can be positioned on armboards at the sides of the bed, as in the prone position, or in anatomic alignment, resting on the bed beneath the abdomen of the patient. Pressure points to be assessed include the eyes, ears, breasts of females, genitalia of males, knees, and toes.

Moving the patient out of the prone or knee-chest position should be accomplished with adequate personnel to prevent injury by moving the patient gently and slowly.

Documentation

Documentation is necessary during all phases of the nursing process, demonstrating accountability for nursing care and actions. It should indicate the level and quality of care provided and the nursing care provisions taken to protect the patient's rights. Documentation specific for the orthopaedic patient includes:

- Operative procedure, preoperative and postoperative diagnosis
- Additional procedure(s)
- Names of persons participating in the procedure
- Operation times
- Counts: instruments, sponges, "sharps" (needles, blades)
- Surgical wound classification
- Disposition of specimens
- Medications administered
- Urinary output and estimated blood loss
- Placement of drains
- Equipment
- Implants

Additional procedures commonly occurring in orthopaedics involve use of radiographs, including x-ray films and fluoroscopy (C-arm). Patient protection, such as leaded shields, should be documented. Documentation of equipment includes use of tourniquets, including time and pressure, and use of electrosurgical units or other items that may require retrieval in the event of a patient care problem.

Documentation of equipment use that may not be included in the permanent patient record includes sterilization results of the biologic monitor in loads containing instruments and implants used for orthopaedic procedures. Implant records are maintained, including the implant name, size, amount used, and lot numbers (if appropriate); the date of the procedure; the name of the surgeon; and the patient's name and number. Documentation requirements are established for each institution. A computerized system can be used for data retrieval and can also serve as a mechanism for ordering supplies on a replacement basis.

Infection Control

Infection control measures to reduce clean wound infections during orthopaedic procedures include maintaining traffic patterns, airflow, and aseptic practices with skin cleansing and the draping procedures or other activities that take place intraoperatively. These must be emphasized because of the potential repercussions associated with infection. The majority of postoperative wound infections are caused by airborne contamination. Patient conditions also increase the risk of developing an infection. Markedly obese patients have an infection rate of 18%; malnourished patients, 22.4%; diabetic patients, 10.4%; and patients taking steroids, 16%. Appropriate measures, including aseptic technique, surgical team discipline, and appropriate use of antibiotics, can reduce infection rates to between 1% and 1.5% (Drez, 1991).

Nursing activities require vigilant monitoring of the environment and personnel actions. Adherence to principles of aseptic technique is the most valuable beginning step to controlling infection for any surgical patient and should be carefully monitored during orthopaedic procedures. In addition, other environmental measures may be taken in orthopaedic procedures, including use of air exhaust systems, body exhaust systems, or other products on the market. Acceptable low rates of clean wound infections can be achieved with continuous, conscientious effort on the part of all team members.

Activities that should be rated as high priority and implemented by the surgical team include:

- Following conscientious practices using universal precautions
- Wearing correct operating room attire properly
- Reducing traffic in and around the room and limiting the number of visitors
- Planning traffic patterns for the surgical procedure to allow access to equipment and movement around the room without compromising the sterile surgical field
- Ensuring minimal talking
- Keeping doors and cabinets closed
- Avoiding procedures on patients with infected skin lesions or active dermatitis
- Maintaining surgical technique with effective hemostasis and gentle handling of tissue
- Double gloving or wearing heavy gloves if forceful contact with instruments is anticipated
- Encouraging preoperative germicidal showers for patients
- Maintaining a clean environment and ensuring that equipment is cleaned following patient use

Maintaining **airflow** in the surgical suite has been determined to be a measure for controlling infections. The development of clean-air operating rooms, in which the incoming air is filtered and rendered virtually free of bacteria, has progressed rapidly since the first report of their use by Charnley and Eftekhar in 1969, specifically for replacement of the hip. The principle of operating in a "bacteria-free" environment is preferred for prevention of infections that are serious and costly following orthopaedic procedures.

Laminar airflow is a special air-handling system for improving the filtration, dilution, and distribution of air. It is a controlled, unidirectional, positive pressure stream of air that moves either horizontally or vertically across the operative area and room. The controlled airstream entrains particulate matter and microorganisms, preventing drifting with uncontrolled movement. The flow returns to the system, passes through a prefilter to remove gross particles, and passes through a high-efficiency particulate air filter that traps and eliminates over 99% of all particles larger than 0.3 μm (McQuarrie, Glover, and Olson, 1990). Even though laminar airflow has been shown to decrease the bacterial count at the surgical site, it is not believed to be necessary if the standard air exchanges per hour occur, positive air pressure is maintained, and antibiotics are administered in a timely manner.

Skin cleansing preoperatively reduces bacteria introduced to the surgical site. Surgeons may request cleansing with an antibacterial solution to decrease bioburden on the skin within 24 hours before the scheduled surgical procedure. Prior to preparation of the surgical site in the operating room, the area should be assessed. If the extremity is the operative site, nails should be cleaned thoroughly. Traumatized areas may require denuding or copious irrigation prior to the surgical preparation. Hair that interferes with the surgical procedure should be removed using a depilatory or razor. Shaving should be done as close to the time of the procedure as possible. If done in the operating room, a wet shave should be required and nicks or cuts prevented.

Agents selected for the surgical preparation should have broad-spectrum, antimicrobial action, should be nontoxic, and should provide long-acting protection. The area prepared should be large enough to avoid wound contamination by movement of the drapes. The site should be prepared in a manner that prevents returning to the incision site. Preparing an extremity requires an assistant to hold the extremity. The assistant holding the extremity should be familiar with aseptic technique to prevent contamination of the area prepared. Areas should be protected from pooling of solutions during the preparation by placing an impervious drape or towels for absorption. Vulnerable areas for pooling are beneath the tourniquet, in the groin, and beneath the patient.

Draping procedures and the type of drape can decrease infection rates. Water-repellent disposable drapes are more effective than linen drapes in preventing migration of bacteria. Adhesive drapes have not demonstrated reduction of infection rates (Drez, 1991) but do prevent migration of bacteria. Adherence to aseptic technique during the draping procedure can be the most cost-effective proven measure for minimizing the possibility of wound infection.

Antibiotics should be administered within an hour before the procedure to reduce infection. If the procedure is on an extremity, an antibiotic should be administered in bolus form approximately 20 minutes before the tourniquet is inflated or the incision is made (Drez, Finney, and Roberts, 1991). A broad-spectrum antibiotic, such as a cephalosporin, is often recommended.

EVALUATION

The perioperative nurse evaluates the patient's progress toward attainment of outcomes. The evaluation process is systematic and ongoing, resulting in changing the plan of care as identified by assessment. Collected data should be compared with outcome criteria to determine the extent of attainment of goals. Verbal and documented communication of findings is also necessary for continuity of care. Evaluation is accomplished immediately following the procedure, in the postoperative area or possibly by contact with the patient postoperatively. The patient care situation determines the appropriate way to complete the evaluation. Information can be used to determine measures that should be implemented to improve care of other patients.

Quality Improvement

Quality improvement is a method of assessing the overall effectiveness of direct and indirect nursing care. The Joint Commission on Accreditation of Healthcare Organizations (JCAHO) encouraged provision of high-quality health services by developing a generic 10-step model to assess patient care outcomes and guide the process that may lead to improved patient care delivery. The Association of Operating Room Nurses has published standards consistent with the JCAHO model (Association of Operating Room Nurses, 1992) (see box).

An emphasis on quality improvement (QI) forms a link between perioperative nurses providing patient care and numerous other individuals involved in the care and aids in achieving a standard of excellence in an objective and comprehensive manner that benefits patients. The orthopaedic service has numerous opportunities for implementing the QI process and specific monitoring for improvements in the specialty area (Williams, Neaton, and Myers, 1991).

Delineation of the scope of patient care activities or services includes the patient population, customers served, clinical care activities, services provided, and physical site. Important aspects of care for the orthopaedic patient population often include high volume,

---

> **AORN quality improvement standards for perioperative nursing**
>
> Standard I: Assign responsibility for monitoring and evaluation activities.
> Standard II: Delineate the scope of patient care activities or services.
> Standard III: Identify important aspects that impact the quality of patient care.
> Standard IV: Identify quality indicators for each important aspect of care.
> Standard V: Establish thresholds for evaluation of indicators.
> Standard VI: Collect and organize data for evaluation.
> Standard VII: Evaluate care based on cumulative data.
> Standard VIII: Take actions to improve care and services.
> Standard IX: Assess the effectiveness of action(s) and document outcomes.
> Standard X: Communicate relevant information to organization-wide, quality assessment program.

From Association of Operating Room Nurses: *Quality improvement in perioperative nursing*, Denver, 1992, AORN.

---

high risk, and/or problem-prone areas requiring attention.

Quality indicators are to be identified for each important aspect of care, focusing on structure, process, and outcome. The indicators must be objective, measurable, and based on current knowledge and clinical experience. The plan should include criteria from Standards for Perioperative Clinical Practice; Standards for Perioperative Administrative Practice; Patient Outcomes: Standards of Perioperative Care; Standards of Perioperative Professional Performance; and AORN Recommended Practices for Perioperative Nursing (Association of Operating Room Nurses, 1993).

Indicators should be independent of each other and should measure appropriate protocols. Criteria are determined for each indicator to further define the data to be collected for the indicator. Data are collected on the indicators and evaluated to determine ongoing needs for improved patient care or areas of improvement. The QI process is ongoing, and the method of data collection is specific for each indicator. The result of ongoing monitoring is improved patient care.

Postoperative Complications

Postoperative complications of surgical procedures, or even poor results, can follow even the best of treatment. The physical nature of orthopaedic procedures sometimes results in complications that are more obvious and often long term. Complications addressed in this section include fat embolism syndrome, thromboembolism, infection, and compartment syndrome.

Fat embolism syndrome is commonly associated with multiple fractures or crush injury. Fat globules are released into the circulation from the marrow and the site of local tissue trauma. These pass through the pulmonary vasculature, lodge in the lung, and embolize the circulation. Fatty acids, produced to eliminate the embolus, are toxic to the pulmonary vascular tree, to lung surfactant's, and to the alveolar structure.

The most common signs and symptoms of fat embolism syndrome are those of adult respiratory distress syndrome (ARDS) in association with musculoskeletal trauma with long-bone fractures and injury to the pelvis, coupled with hypovolemia and the development of early respiratory distress. Following fracture, 60% of patients exhibit signs and symptoms within 24 hours and 85% by 48 hours. The remainder of patients show clinically apparent signs and symptoms by the third to the fifth postoperative day. Oxygen desaturation, fever, and sinus tachycardia constitute a triad of early findings. Multisystem effects include an alteration of mental status ranging from drowsiness, restlessness, and mild irritability to confusion, disorientation, stupor, and coma.

Clinical signs and symptoms associated with the fat embolism syndrome are evident in 0.5% to 2% of patients with long-bone fractures and in nearly 10% of patients with multiple skeletal fractures associated with unstable pelvic injuries, although the syndrome can occur following many orthopaedic procedures (Gossling and Pellegrini, 1982). It has been estimated that on an annual basis more than 5000 deaths are directly caused by the fat embolism syndrome (Evarts, 1990). Current therapy is parenteral cortisone, and reversal of the life-threatening hypoxemia and acute respiratory failure associated with fat embolism. Most recent literature has focused on the role of early operative fracture stabilization in preventing the development of the pulmonary complications associated with posttraumatic fat embolism.

It has been difficult to ascribe a direct casual relationship to intravascular pulmonary fat seen on postmortem examination. It is generally agreed that bone marrow is the source of embolic fat in the production of the clinical fat embolism syndrome. It has also become increasingly apparent that embolic marrow fat and other elements are an early link in a long chain of events leading to increased pulmonary vascular permeability in response to many forms of systemic injury.

Thromboembolic disease (deep venous thrombosis and thromboembolism) is one of the most common and dangerous of all complications occurring after skeletal trauma and elective musculoskeletal surgery. It may develop as the result of vessel wall injury, local venous stasis, and the release of factors that activate the coagulation system. An estimated 150,000 deaths annually in the United States are attributed to thromboembolic disease (Evarts, 1990). The threat of this disease is correlated with age, obesity, the extent and duration of the musculoskeletal procedure, the degree and length of immobilization, a past history of thromboembolic disease, and the severity of the underlying systemic disease.

In orthopaedics venous thrombosis is reported in 45% to 70% of the patient population undergoing total hip or knee replacement, hip fracture, and major knee reconstruction (Concensus, 1986). The exact sequence of events leading to thrombus formation after skeletal trauma or musculoskeletal surgery is not completely understood. Initiating mechanisms are obscure, clinical recognition is elusive, the recurrence rate is high, and the mortality rate is unpredictable. Signs and symptoms of deep venous thrombosis are unreliable, but commonly pain, deep tenderness, swelling, and redness of the extremity should be evaluated. The detection of venous thrombosis cannot be based on these findings alone, because at least two thirds are silent and never detected clinically.

Prevention of venous thromboembolic disease includes maintenance of fluid and electrolyte balance and prevention of shock. Following loss of blood or fluids, replacement therapy must be adequate to avoid dehydration. The management of the surgical or traumatic wound is important. Surgical time should be as brief as possible. All associated illnesses must be identified and appropriate treatment instituted. The nutritional status of the patient must be closely evaluated and monitored, with correction occurring when necessary. Intraoperatively it may be necessary to begin anticoagulant therapy.

In the early postoperative or postinjury period, the patient must be encouraged to perform leg—including calf and ankle—movements, with emphasis on the quadriceps, hip musculature, and hamstring contractions. It is important to begin early mobilization of the patient, including active and passive motion of the lower extremity and walking exercises. The foot of the bed should be elevated. The use of thigh-length compression stockings has been shown to aid in postoperative prevention of deep venous thrombosis. It has been suggested, but not proved, that continuous passive motion may prevent deep venous thrombosis in the postoperative patient.

Antiplatelet agents and anticoagulants have been demonstrated to prevent thromboemboli. Because of the multifactorial nature of venous thromboembolism, it is thought that combination therapy, including both antiplatelet and antithrombotic agents, may be more effective than single agents.

Pulmonary embolism is one of the most serious, underdiagnosed (and often fatal) complications facing the orthopaedist today. Ninety percent of pulmonary emboli arise from deep venous thrombosis. The most common clinical manifestations are sudden apprehension, dyspnea, tachycardia, and rales. Patients also feel an urgent need to go to the bathroom because of the dilation of hemorrhoidal veins. Because pulmonary embolism is related to deep venous thrombosis, there is a strong need for early recognition, preventive measures, and immediate treatment once the embolism occurs.

Wound infection has been estimated by the American College of Surgeons to cost an average of $6000 to $900,000 and to result in 80,000 deaths annually (Drez, Finney, and Roberts, 1991). Infections following bone and joint procedures can be devastating, resulting in a stiff, painful joint; the need to remove an implant; long-bone drains; and failure to unite.

Orthopaedic infections can be evaluated from two aspects: (1) infection that occurs because of the orthopaedic condition or procedure and (2) complications that arise following a musculoskeletal infection. Causes may be patient dependent or technique dependent. Patient-dependent factors include nutritional status, immunologic status, and infection at a remote site. Endogenous infections spread from a septic focus such as poor dentition, urinary tract infection, or a local infection. Technique-dependent factors include use of prophylactic antibiotics, skin and wound care, operating room environment, surgical technique, and treatment of impending infections.

Postoperatively, infections may present as persistent, unexplained pain; effusion; erythema; prolonged drainage from the wound; and failure of primary wound healing. An elevated white blood cell count (WBC) may only be present in fulminating infections; therefore a normal WBC does not exclude infection. Superficial wound infections can progress to deep infections and can result in osteomylitis or septic arthritis.

Bacterial osteomylitis is a suppurative process in bone caused by a pyogenic organism. It may remain localized or may spread through the bone to involve marrow, cortex, periosteum, and soft tissue. Symptoms may be severe pain, bone tenderness, high fever, headache, and vomiting, although patients usually have vague symptoms with an insidious onset. Early detection and treatment of infection is the key to preventing chronic osteomylitis and osseous destruction.

Compartment syndrome is described as increased pressure compromising the circulation and function of tissue. The compartment consists of bone, blood vessels, nerves, muscle, and soft tissue. Those compartments most commonly involved include the forearm and leg, although any area is at risk for this complication. Symptoms of compartment syndrome include hypesthesia, weakness, pain on stretching the muscles, and abnormal pain for the type of injury. Peripheral pulses are not usually affected. If medical interventions are not effective, a fasciotomy with irrigation and debridement will be necessary. The incision(s) are packed open following debridement.

BIBLIOGRAPHY

AMA Council on Scientific Affairs: High risk profile for elder abuse and neglect, *JAMA* 257:966, 1987.

American Nurses Association: *Standards of clinical nursing practice*, Kansas City, 1991, American Nurses Association.

Association of Operating Room Nurses: *Quality improvement in perioperative nursing*, Denver, 1992, AORN.

Association of Operating Room Nurses: *AORN standards and recommended practices for perioperative nursing—1993*, Denver, 1993, AORN.

Barangan J: Factors that influence recovery from hip fractures during hospitalization, *Orthop Nurs* 9:19, Sept/Oct 1990.

Barnes CL, Blasier RD, Dodge BM: Intravenous regional anesthesia: a safe and cost-effective outpatient anesthetic for upper extremity fracture treatment in children, *J Pediatr* 11:717, 1991.

Barrett J, Bryant BH: Fractures: types, treatment, perioperative implications, *AORN J* 52:755, Oct 1990.

Biddle C, Cannady M: Surgical positions, their effects on cardiovascular, respiratory systems, *AORN J* 52:350, Aug 1990.

Booth B, Kumar A: Surgery for elderly patients: a new specialty? *Nurs Times* 85:26, July 1989.

Concensus Conference: Prevention of venous thrombosis and pulmonary embolism, *JAMA* 256:744, 1986.

Connolly ML: Ambulatory surgery and prepared discharge: effects on orthopedic patients and nursing practice, *Nurs Clin North Am* 26:105, March 1991.

Drez D, Finney TP, Roberts TS: Sepsis on orthopedic surgery, *Orthopedics* 14:157, Feb 1991.

Evarts CM: *Surgery of the musculoskeletal system*, ed 2, New York, 1990, Churchill Livingstone.

Ferraro KF: *Gerontology: perspectives and issues*, New York, 1990, Springer.

Gordon M: Restoring functional independence in the older hip fracture patient, *Geriatrics* 44:48, Dec 1989.

Gossling HR, Pellegrini VD: Fat embolism syndrome: a review of the pathophysiology and physiological basis of treatment, *Clin Orthop* 165:68, 1982.

Gravenstein N: Anesthesia for joint surgery replacement. In Petty W, editor: *Total joint replacement*, Philadelphia, 1991, WB Saunders/Harcourt Brace Jovanovich.

Groah L: *Operating room nursing, perioperative practice*, ed 2, Norwalk, Conn, 1990, Appleton & Lange.

Hampel G: Closed interlocking nailing in the lower extremity: indications and positioning, *AORN J* 47:1203, May 1988.

Hansell MJ: Fractures and the healing process, *Orthop Nurs* 7:43, Jan/Feb 1988.

Hester R, Nelson C: Current concepts review, methods to reduce intraoperative transmission of blood-borne disease, *J Bone Joint Surg* 73A:1108, Aug 1991.

Magee D: *Orthopedic physical assessment*, Philadelphia, 1987, WB Saunders.

Malawer MM and others: Postoperative infusional continuous regional analgesia: a technique for relief of postoperative pain following major extremity surgery, *Clin Orthop,* 266:227, 1991.

Martin JT: *Positioning in anesthesia and surgery,* ed 2, Philadelphia, 1987, WB Saunders.

McQuarrie DG, Glover JL, Olson M: Laminar airflow systems: issues surrounding their effectiveness, *AORN J* 51:1035, Nov 1990.

Meeker M, Rothrock J: *Alexander's care of the patient in surgery,* ed 9, St Louis, 1991, Mosby.

Mourad LA: *Orthopedic disorders,* St Louis, 1991, Mosby.

Nelson L and others: Improving pain management for hip fractured elderly, *Orthop Nurs* 9:79, May/June 1990.

Orr PM: An educational program for total hip and knee replacement patients as part of a total arthritis center program, *Orthop Nurs* 9:61, Sept/Oct 1990.

Piasecki P, Gitelis S: Use of a clean air system and personal exhaust suit in the orthopaedic operating room, *Orthop Nurs* 7:20, July/Aug 1988.

Ritter MA, Marmion P: The exogenous sources and controls of microorganisms in the operating room, *Orthop Nurs* 7:23, 1988.

Rothrock J: *Perioperative nursing care planning,* St Louis, 1990, Mosby.

Sculco T: *Orthopaedic care of the geriatric patient,* St Louis, 1985, Mosby.

Slye D: Orthopedic complications, compartment syndrome, fat embolism syndrome, and venous thromboembolism, *Orthop Nurs* 26:113, March 1991.

Smith KA: Positioning principles, an anatomical review, *AORN J* 52:1196, Dec 1990.

Smith TK: Nutrition: its relationship to orthopedic infections, *Orthop Clin North Am* 22:373, July 1991.

Touloukian, RN: *Pediatric trauma,* ed 2, St Louis, 1990, Mosby.

Vermillion C: Operating room acquired pressure ulcers, *Decubitus* 3:26, Feb 1990.

Wells M: *Decision making in perioperative nursing,* Toronto, 1987, BC Decker.

Williams NH, Neaton M, Myers S: A quality assurance plan for an epidural analgesia program, *Orthop Nurs* 10:45, May/June 1991.

Zuckerman JD: *Comprehensive care of orthopaedic injuries in the elderly,* Baltimore, 1990, Urban & Schwarzenberg.

5

Instrumentation

Instruments used for orthopaedic procedures continually increase in quantity and sophistication. The budget required for any operating room that does orthopaedic procedures is large, not only because of the expense of each item, but also because of the continual need to update and repair equipment. Perioperative nurses cannot function effectively in this specialty area without understanding the armamentarium of instruments in their clinical focus. Procedures scheduled require an understanding of each patient as an individual in order to determine the appropriate instrumentation. In addition, as the perioperative nurse manages patient care, an awareness of the function, maintenance, troubleshooting, and handling of these instruments is required in order to provide quality care. Instruments used in orthopaedic surgical procedures are discussed in this chapter.

CARE AND HANDLING

Orthopaedic procedures do not differ from other procedures in the need for functional instruments to achieve an effective, safe surgical outcome. Instruments range from delicate to sturdy and must accommodate procedures on varied anatomic structures. Familiarity with these structures will assist personnel in selecting appropriate-size instruments for a particular procedure. During the procedure the correct instrument should be used for the specific purpose for which it has been designed. Improper use results in instru-

ments becoming nonfunctional for other procedures. Examples of misuse that causes damage include:

- Towel clips used to manipulate bone, hemostats used to grab tissue masses or bone, or scissors used to cut wire
- Instruments substituted because one of the correct size and type is not available on the field
- Failure to check instruments routinely for damage and need for sharpening or replacement

Tissue is generally tough and fibrous, requiring instruments that can serve the intended purpose without being damaged. Surgeons expect instruments of the appropriate size and type to be available. Damaged instruments are expensive to repair or replace and result in unsafe patient care.

Instruments properly used and cared for can be expected to remain functional for many years. Proper cleaning of instruments (during surgery, if possible, and following the procedure) helps to prevent stiff joints, malfunction, and deterioration of stainless steel. During surgery instruments contaminated with blood or tissue should be rinsed and wiped with distilled water. Saline should not be used for this purpose, since it can cause corrosion and eventual pitting. Blood and other foreign matter that is allowed to dry and harden may become trapped in jaw serrations between scissors blades or in box locks. This renders the instrument unsterile and can also result in malfunction and corrosion. Tubular instruments, such as drill guides and flexible reamer shafts, should be rinsed immediately. Damage can be avoided by ensuring that instruments are not tangled or stacked with heavy instruments on top of lighter-weight or delicate instruments.

Instruments in Figs. 5-2 through 5-21 are shown by courtesy of Zimmer, Inc.

All instruments placed on the sterile field are to be considered contaminated and should be cleaned promptly. If it is not possible to clean instruments immediately, they should be completely submerged in a container of warm water with detergent until they can be placed in the washer-sterilizer for initial cleaning. Orthopaedic instruments usually require attention to remove blood and debris before they are placed in the washer-sterilizer. Following placement in the washer-sterilizer, the instruments should be placed in the ultrasonic cleaner to remove debris from every part of the instrument and then rinsed.

Inspection of orthopaedic instruments is critical for maintenance. Box locks, joint movement, jaw alignment, and ratchet function should be checked. The instrument should open and close easily. Instruments should not be packaged if they are stained, rusting, or pitted; these are the symptoms of a damaged instrument and should be corrected before use.

BASIC INSTRUMENTS

Basic and specialty instrument sets are organized to accommodate anatomic structures such as large bones, small bones, or extremities. The number and type of instruments placed in the sets are determined by the procedures most commonly scheduled in the operating room. Some instruments used for orthopaedic procedures are heavy; therefore attention must be paid to the total weight of the orthopaedic sets and to the combination of instruments placed in the sets. The maximum weight recommendation of 16 pounds is a factor in determining the amount and type of instruments placed in a set (Association of Operating Room Nurses, 1992).

Basic soft tissue instruments (Fig. 5-1) are needed for incision, soft tissue dissection, and closure. The set should include appropriate sizes, types, and numbers of instruments to meet anatomic needs and surgeon preference. Examples include:

Knife handles: No. 4, No. 3
Scissors: dissecting, suture, bandage
Suction tips: Yankauer, Frazier
Needle holders: Hegar
Towel clips
Retractors: Army-Navy, Senn, Weitlaner, Gelpi
Hemostats
Oschner clamp
Allis clamps
Tissue forceps: Adson, Mayo—with and without teeth

Limiting the potentially large number of instruments on the sterile field will improve the ability of the scrub person to organize the field and maintain awareness of instruments during and following the

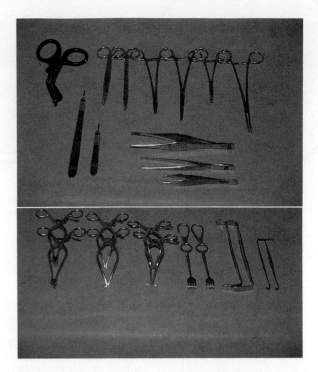

Fig. 5-1   Basic soft tissue instruments.

procedure, preventing inadvertent loss. A soft tissue set for procedures on extremities including the digits, hand, wrist, toes, feet, and ankle would include instruments of appropriate size for the anatomy. Soft tissue sets can also be organized to include small-bone instruments for procedures on the lower arm or leg and other small bones or large-bone instruments for procedures on the upper arm and leg. Large-bone and small-bone instrument sets include the specialty holding, cutting, and retracting instruments for orthopaedic procedures. Discussion of a variety of instruments and their uses follows.

CUTTING INSTRUMENTS

Sharp instruments are used for bone or tissue, in sizes appropriate for small- or large-bone procedures.

An **osteotome** is symmetrically tapered to be used for driving straight into a bone or for dividing the bone to shave or cut it. It is applicable only for cutting bone that is fairly soft, especially cancellous bone or the long bones of children. If the shaft of a long bone must be divided in an adult, it may be necessary to weaken the cortex with multiple drill holes before using the osteotome. Osteotomes range in width from smaller than ¼ inch to 1 inch or wider and are straight or curved. Small, delicate osteotomes are used for hand or foot procedures. The osteotome is requested by size and curvature.

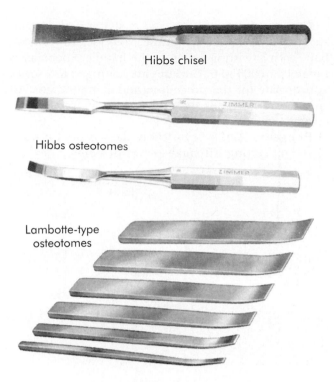

Hibbs chisel

Hibbs osteotomes

Lambotte-type osteotomes

Fig. 5-2   Osteotomes and chisel.

Chisels and osteotomes (Fig. 5-2) are used for taking shavings or smoothing off irregularities to prepare a flat surface to receive a plate or bone graft. They are designed to be used with mallets. A chisel is beveled only on one side, and it is important that it be held in the correct direction for the desired function. When shavings are taken from a flat surface, the beveled side should be held toward the bone. For smoothing a convex surface, the chisel is held with the flat surface against the bone. The same position is used for cutting a notch or groove in a bone.

Gouges (Fig. 5-3) are more suitable than chisels for working on rounded concavities such as the acetabulum or iliac crest. They are designed to scoop bone away and are used primarily to harvest bone grafts and prepare bone for receiving bone graft. A narrow gouge is useful for making a notch as the starting point for a drill or for countersinking a screw.

Elevators (Fig. 5-4) are chisel-like instruments with rounded tips designed to elevate periosteum and muscle fibers from the bone without cutting the bone.

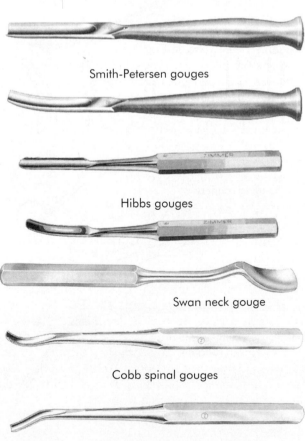

Smith-Petersen gouges

Hibbs gouges

Swan neck gouge

Cobb spinal gouges

Fig. 5-3   Gouges.

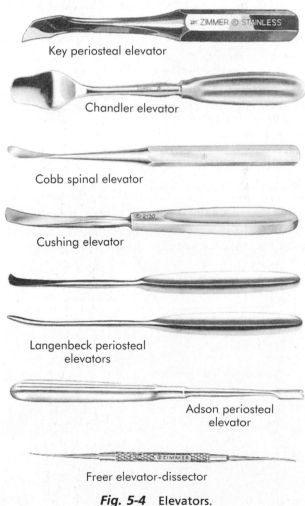

Key periosteal elevator

Chandler elevator

Cobb spinal elevator

Cushing elevator

Langenbeck periosteal elevators

Adson periosteal elevator

Freer elevator-dissector

Fig. 5-4   Elevators.

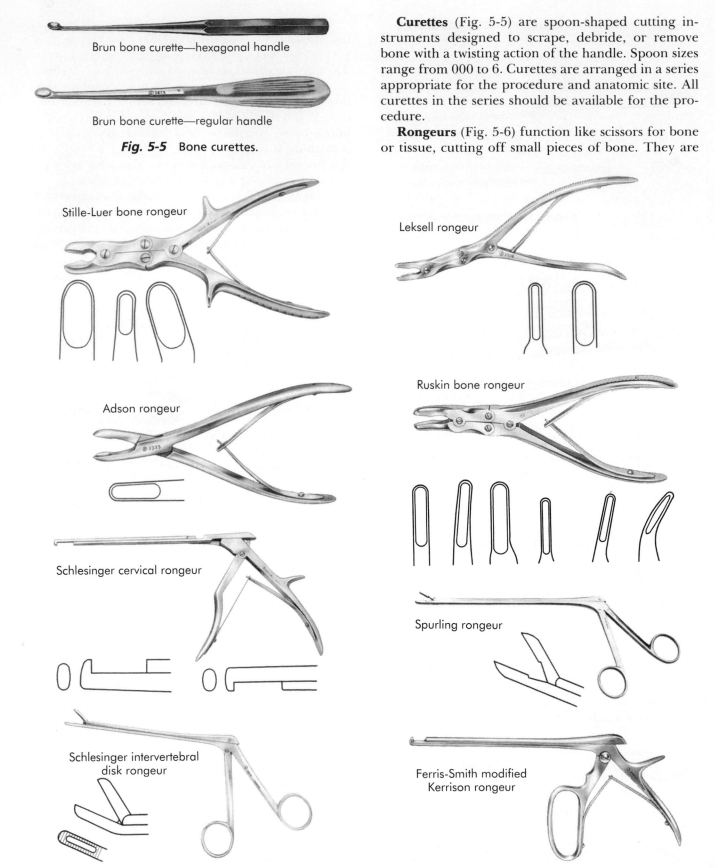

Brun bone curette—hexagonal handle

Brun bone curette—regular handle

Fig. 5-5   Bone curettes.

Curettes (Fig. 5-5) are spoon-shaped cutting instruments designed to scrape, debride, or remove bone with a twisting action of the handle. Spoon sizes range from 000 to 6. Curettes are arranged in a series appropriate for the procedure and anatomic site. All curettes in the series should be available for the procedure.

Rongeurs (Fig. 5-6) function like scissors for bone or tissue, cutting off small pieces of bone. They are

Stille-Luer bone rongeur

Leksell rongeur

Adson rongeur

Ruskin bone rongeur

Schlesinger cervical rongeur

Spurling rongeur

Schlesinger intervertebral disk rongeur

Ferris-Smith modified Kerrison rongeur

Fig. 5-6   Rongeurs.

available in over 20 different types. The cutting end resembles a double set of opposed curettes. A double-action rongeur has two hinge joints; a single-action rongeur has only one. A moistened sponge is used to remove the bone or tissue from the rongeur. The size of rongeur selected will depend on the anatomic structure.

Bone-cutting forceps (Fig. 5-7) are available in double action or single action. Single-action forceps are more precise and useful for small- or soft-bone work. They function more effectively when bone is placed in the depth of the jaw. Both sides of the bone must be stabilized when forceps are used.

Bone rasps (Fig. 5-8) are available for smoothing and shaping bone surfaces or evacuating the medullary canal for insertion of a stemmed prosthesis. They come in many sizes and shapes.

BONE-HOLDING INSTRUMENTS

Instruments for holding bones (Fig. 5-9) are available for large-bone or small-bone procedures. They are used to grasp fragmented bone and hold it in place for application of a fixating device or for holding a plate during fixation. Bone holders are usually self-retaining, which means they have a dual-lock mechanism that secures the forceps to the bone until fixation is applied. They are usually used in pairs. Bone hooks are used for retraction and leverage of bone fragments.

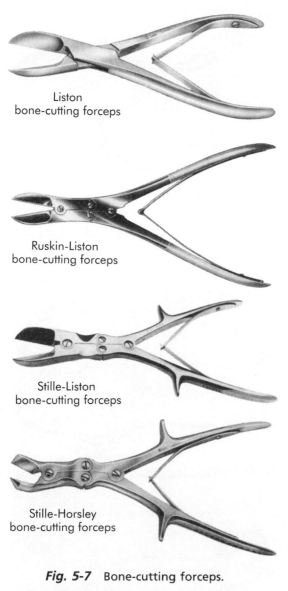

Fig. 5-7 Bone-cutting forceps.

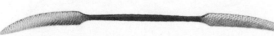

Fig. 5-8 Double-ended Putti bone rasp.

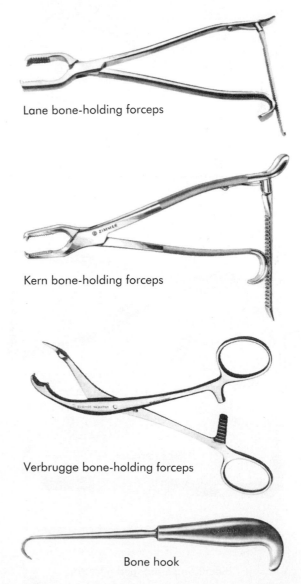

Fig. 5-9 Bone-holding forceps, bone hook, and clamps.

Continued.

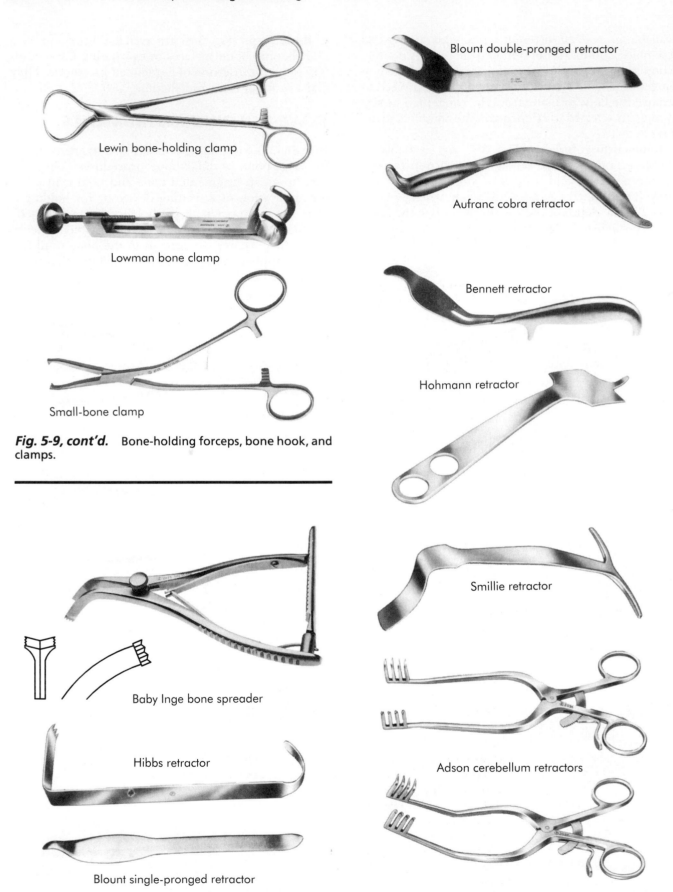

Lewin bone-holding clamp

Lowman bone clamp

Small-bone clamp

Blount double-pronged retractor

Aufranc cobra retractor

Bennett retractor

Hohmann retractor

Fig. 5-9, cont'd. Bone-holding forceps, bone hook, and clamps.

Baby Inge bone spreader

Hibbs retractor

Blount single-pronged retractor

Smillie retractor

Adson cerebellum retractors

Fig. 5-10 Bone spreader and retractors.

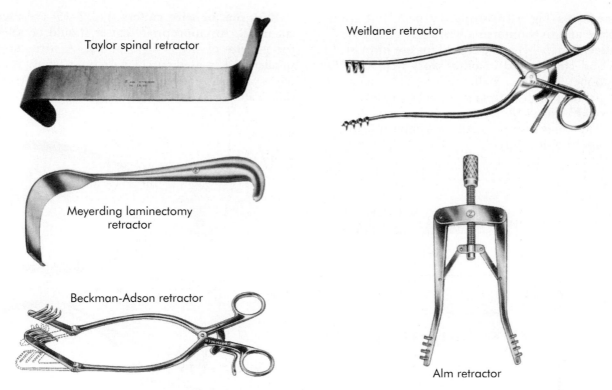

Taylor spinal retractor

Weitlaner retractor

Meyerding laminectomy retractor

Beckman-Adson retractor

Alm retractor

Fig. 5-10, cont'd. Bone spreader and retractors.

RETRACTING INSTRUMENTS

Soft tissue retraction is accomplished with instruments commonly used in other specialties in addition to special bone retraction instruments (Fig. 5-10). Orthopaedic retractors are designed to bear against bone while atraumatically retracting the soft tissue.

NONSPECIFIC CATEGORIES

Many instruments are used in orthopaedic procedures that are not included in basic categories. These are described according to their name or function.

Plate benders and **bending pliers** (Fig. 5-11) are used for gently shaping a plate to fit the patient. They should not be used to angle a plate because one of the correct shape is not available. Plates should not be bent forward and backwards which causes weakening. If reverse bending takes place, the plate should be discarded.

Bone awls (Fig. 5-12) are used for perforating cancellous bone and thin cortical bone when a drill is not useful or desired.

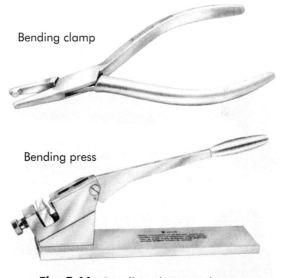

Bending clamp

Bending press

Fig. 5-11 Bending clamp and press.

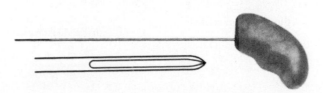

Fig. 5-12 Rush awl reamer.

Bone tamps (Fig. 5-13) are used to pack bone grafts into place and to countersink wires.

Mallets (Fig. 5-14) are designed for use with osteotomes and chisels, and in other work that requires metal-to-metal contact. Mallets are available in small and large sizes, are usually composed of stainless steel, and should be available for most orthopaedic procedures. They may also be made of Teflon for procedures requiring less force.

Rod, pin, or wire cutters (Fig. 5-15) are used to cut metal. An appropriate cutter should be selected for the size of the item to be cut. A wire cutter is smaller and is used to cut Kirschner wires. Cutting pliers can also be used to trim unnecessary parts from thin plates.

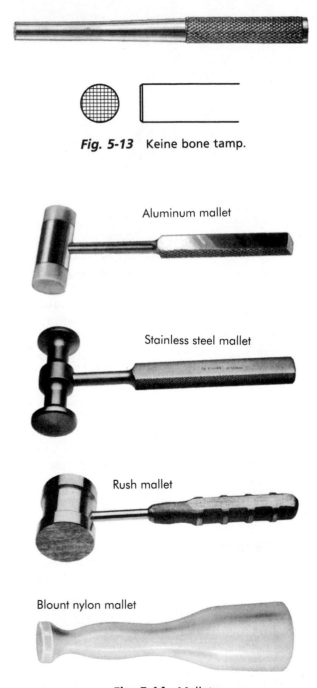

Fig. 5-13   Keine bone tamp.

Aluminum mallet

Stainless steel mallet

Rush mallet

Blount nylon mallet

Fig. 5-14   Mallets.

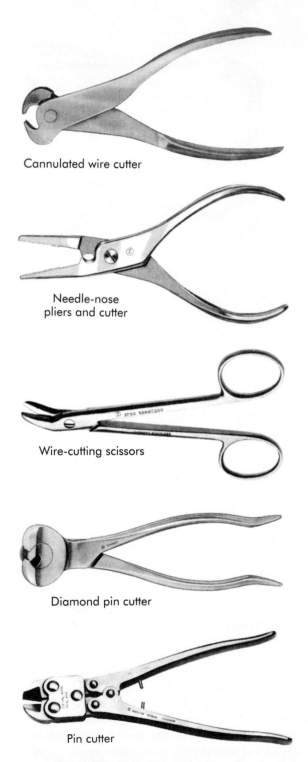

Cannulated wire cutter

Needle-nose
pliers and cutter

Wire-cutting scissors

Diamond pin cutter

Pin cutter

Fig. 5-15   Rod, pin, and wire cutters.

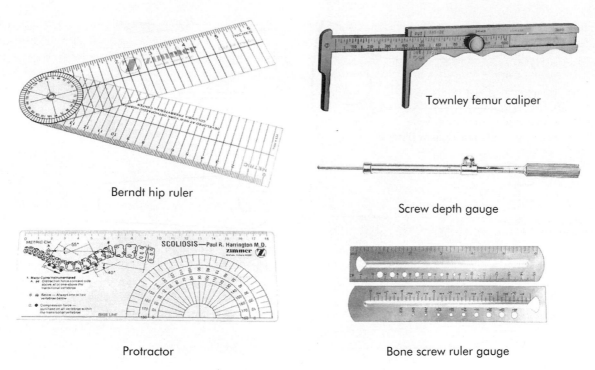

Berndt hip ruler

Townley femur caliper

Screw depth gauge

Protractor

Bone screw ruler gauge

Fig. 5-16 Measuring devices.

Measuring devices (Fig. 5-16) include calipers, depth gauges, rulers, and goniometers. A caliper is used to measure the width of an anatomic part, such as the femoral head, when a prosthesis is to be inserted. A depth gauge is used to measure the depth of a hole made by the drill bit. A ruler is used for several purposes, including measuring screw length.

Screwdrivers are commonly used to insert or remove a screw through a plate or bone. The screwdriver may be power driven or manually operated. They are available in Phillips, cross-slot, single-slot, and hexagonal heads. Screwdrivers with damaged tips should not be used; they would damage the socket in the screw head, making it difficult or impossible to remove the screw.

Pliers are multipurpose instruments used in orthopaedic procedures. They should not be used to repair instruments.

Power-driven instruments are available in many sizes and design. Chucks are heads that allow the use of tools of different sizes. A chuck key is used with a Jacobs or universal chuck; it is inserted in the chuck to increase or decrease the diameter of the hole in the chuck to accept the variously sized drill bits to be used. Precautions that should be taken when operating power equipment include avoiding:

- Pointing the drill or loaded handpiece in the direction of a team member when it is activated
- Handing a loaded drill to the surgeon before testing it

- Leaving a drill on the sterile field where it may be activated accidentally
- Using the drill without providing saline irrigation to prevent the bone from overheating
- Using power equipment without eye protection

Compressed air equipment provides the ability to drill, ream, and saw. A handpiece, hose, and supplementary attachments are standard parts of this equipment. Nitrogen is commonly supplied in a cylinder or by a continuous source piped into the operating room. The compressed air equipment requires special handling by the scrub and circulating personnel. The supply of air should be assessed to determine that an adequate amount is available. If air cylinders are used, the cylinder quantity for screw/plate fixation should be a minimum of 3000 pounds per square inch (psi) with about 6000 psi for reaming. The contents should not drop below 500 psi during a procedure. Operating hoses should be checked for leaks and function when connected, before the incision is made. During use or storage the hoses should not be kinked or woven tightly. The speed of the drill is controlled with a trigger or footpedal. A control for forward, reverse, and safety is usually found on the handpiece. Power-driven equipment can also be operated with a specialized battery. An adequate supply of batteries should be available for several procedures, and battery packs must be checked to ensure that they are charged. When the power drill is used, onward pressure should be controlled at all times as a safeguard

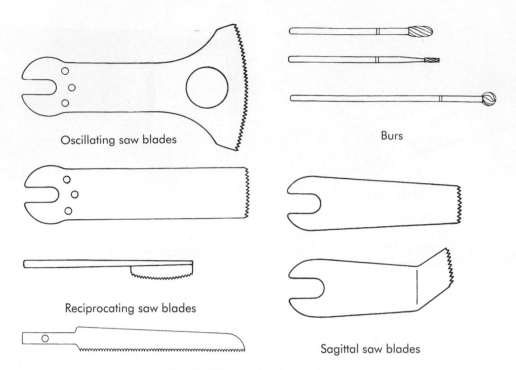

Oscillating saw blades

Burs

Reciprocating saw blades

Sagittal saw blades

Fig. 5-17 Saw blades and burs.

against inadvertent damage to a structure by penetration of the drill.

Blades and burs (Fig. 5-17) are available for power-driven equipment to accomplish precise transverse or longitudinal cuts for the surgical procedure. Blades and burs have limited lives. If disposables are used, they should be discarded following each procedure.

Burs rotate at very high speeds and are useful for fine work on bones such as those in the hands and feet and the laminae of the spine. A range of burs is available for cutting and drilling. A revolving bur is used for cutting in the manner of a fine knife. Most cutting burs may also be used for drilling soft bone.

An oscillating saw blade cuts by moving through a small arc. Cutting is achieved by pressing the blade vertically against the bone, section by section rather than by moving it along the bone continuously. The reciprocating saw blade is used by applying steady pressure to engage the teeth of the saw in the bone without moving the body of the saw while maintaining a view of the tip of the saw blade throughout the sawing process.

Manual drilling can be accomplished with relative ease, since even hard bone can be penetrated provided that the drill bit is sharp. A hand drill (Fig. 5-18) can be used for all purposes except sawing. Standard applications include insertion of wires or pins, drilling, tapping, and screw insertion or removal and reaming.

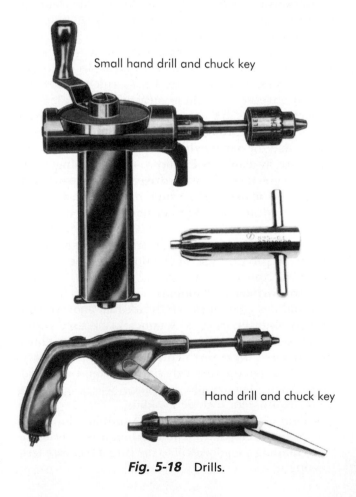

Small hand drill and chuck key

Hand drill and chuck key

Fig. 5-18 Drills.

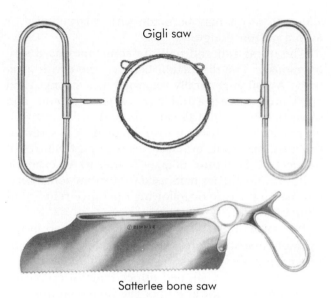

Gigli saw

Satterlee bone saw

Fig. 5-19 Saws.

Manual, or hand, saws (Fig. 5-19) include amputation saws and Gigli saws. An amputation saw is used for entirely dividing bone during amputation of a limb. A Gigli saw is a flexible wire with cutting teeth arranged in spirals on the circumference. Operation of the Gigli saw requires use of Gigli saw handles. One end of the saw is passed around the deep surface of the bone, and an end is held in each hand by the handle. The saw is worked with a reciprocal action.

Orthopedic implants include prostheses, plates, screws, nails, rods, staples, wires, and pins for fixation, temporary stabilization, or permanent replacement of bone, joints, or tendons. The substance used for manufacturing these implants is selected for strength and inert qualities. Decisions about use of cobalt-chrome alloy, stainless steel, titanium, silicone, or polyethylene or polytetrafluroethylene implants are made by the physician scheduling the procedure. Operating room personnel are expected to maintain adequate supplies of implants. Implants of different types and origin are not interchangeable. Also, they should not be reused if exposed to stressful conditions. Unstressed implants (a screw replaced during a procedure because of incorrect length) may be reused. Contouring and bending of implants is discouraged, since it may reduce fatigue strength and cause either immediate or eventual failure under load.

Manufactured implants are extremely expensive and should be handled with care. Polished areas should not come in contact with hard or abrasive surfaces. Once an implant has been scratched or damaged, it cannot be used; therefore care must be taken when storing and handling implants. Many implants are prepackaged by the manufacturer. As with all packages, they should be inspected for damage before being opened. If the implant is not packaged sterilely but responsibility for sterilization is assumed by hospital personnel, a biologic monitor should be run in the load with the implant. The biologic monitor provides assurance that the sterilizer parameters were met during the cycle.

Materials used for total joint replacement prostheses include naturally occurring metals and their alloys. The development of alloys with increased mechanical strength has improved the outcome of total joint procedures. Computer-assisted design and machining systems are intended to provide improved patient anatomic compatibility. These specialized implants also affect implant availability and procedure planning.

Screws are used to hold bones together, to hold appliances to the bone until natural healing has occurred, or to secure tendons and ligaments. Screws are made of inert metal; therefore it is not always necessary to remove them. Screws cannot be expected to serve holding purposes permanently. If natural healing fails to occur, a screw will eventually loosen or break. Screws usually are made from cobalt-chromium alloy or special (18/8 SMo) stainless steel. Screws are plain or self-tapping. The screw selected will depend on the hardness or softness of the bone. The cortex of long bones in adults is hard. All cancellous bone, as well as the cortex of flat bones and the cortex of long bones in young children, is softer. Hard bone will not accept a screw unless the drill hole made to receive it is tapped with matching threads. Soft bone will take a screw without tapping and often without predrilling. To drive a screw into the adult cortical bone, a hole equal in diameter to the root diameter of the screw must always be drilled and the hole must either be tapped or a self-tapping screw must be used. In cancellous bone, the receiving hole is undersized and a cross-slot rather than a self-tapping screw may be used if desired. Types of screws (Fig. 5-20) include:

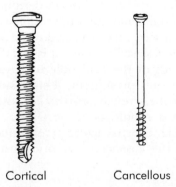

Cortical   Cancellous

Fig. 5-20 Cortical and cancellous screws (partially threaded).

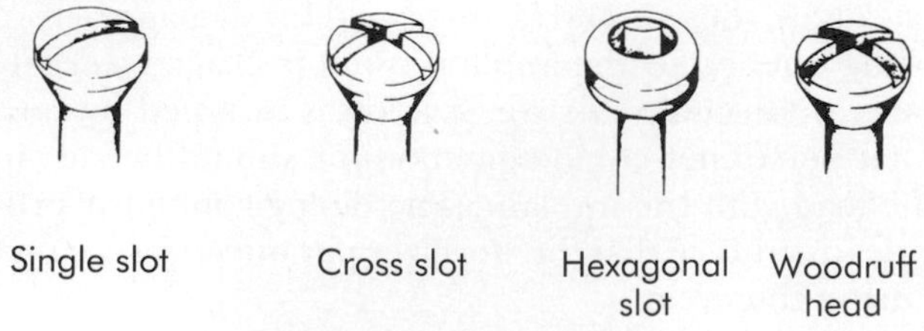

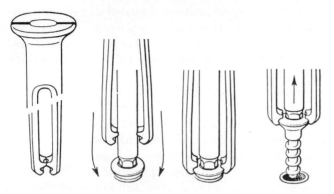

Single slot   Cross slot   Hexagonal   Woodruff
                              slot   head

Fig. 5-21 Screw heads.

Fig. 5-22 **Screwdriver with holding sleeve used for placing screws.** (From Heim U, Pfeiffer KM: *Internal fixation of small fractures,* ed 3, New York, 1988, Springer-Verlag.)

- Cortex screws: fully threaded; designed for hard cortical bone
- Cancellous bone and malleolar screws: partially threaded with a smooth shaft

Screw length is measured for verification prior to placement; the length includes the head when measured. A cross-slot screw (Fig. 5-21) can be used with a cross-head screwdriver. Screws with a cruciform recess of Phillips pattern are used with a Phillips screwdriver. The screws designed by the Swiss Association of Osteosynthesis (AO) have a hexagonal recess for use with a special screwdriver (Fig. 5-22).

Most screws have tapered heads designed for countersinking. Metal plates and other appliances are supplied with recessed holes to receive the screw heads. When bone is screwed to bone, it is usual to countersink the mouth of the drill hole to ensure that the screw head is not prominent. This is an important precaution if the screw head is to lie close under the skin. Recessing should be done with a countersink made to match the particular screws that are to be used, but in the absence of such an instrument, an adequate recess may be made with a larger drill or even a narrow gouge.

The terms **rod** and **nail** are sometimes used synonymously. The distinction between the two is arbitrary. A nail is generally regarded as a strong, rigid appliance, whereas a rod is much more slender and often to some extent flexible. Smooth nails and rods do not have the friction to hold, as does a screw or threaded pin. Nails are used for fixating fractures of the neck of the femur, tibia, or humerus. An example is the intramedullary nails used for fixating long bones to repair a fracture or following operative removal of a tumor or cyst.

Pins of more slender proportions are used in the form of Kirschner wires (K-wires) or Steinmann pins for the purpose of fixating bone fragments (i.e., in the treatment of a slipped upper femoral epiphysis, a fracture of the lower end of the fibula, an unstable fracture of the metacarpal shaft, and certain fractures and dislocations of the clavicle). Pins can be used for purposes varying from transfixing a long bone to applying skeletal traction. Pins used for these purposes are sometimes threaded or partly threaded. An absorbable pin is available for the fixation of small bony or chondral fragments where rapid healing is anticipated and fragments are not under tension. The advantages are that pin site infection is minimized and stability is maintained until the pin absorbs.

Staples are a useful method of internal fixation of soft bone. A staple may be placed at a site composed of cancellous bone, such as in maintaining opposition of the tarsal bones after osteotomy, or as an aid to achieving tarsal arthrodesis. Stapling is also standard for fixation after a wedge osteotomy of the upper end of the tibia for correction of genu varum or genu valgum. Wide staples give a better grip than narrow ones, but the width that can be used is often restricted by the proximity of adjacent joints or other structures. Staple length is critical and dependent on sufficient available bone depth. A staple starter of matching size is hammered in to prepare the holes for the legs of the staple. An automatic staple gun can also be used.

Wire is used to secure bone fragments together or to secure muscle, tendon, or ligament to bone. Wire sutures are used for attaching tendon or muscle to bone in a variety of situations. Examples are reattachment of the quadriceps tendon to the upper pole of the patella in the repair of traumatic avulsion and attachment of the triceps muscle to the stump of the olecranon after excision of the olecranon process for treatment of a comminuted fracture.

BIBLIOGRAPHY

Association of Operating Room Nurses: *AORN standards and recommended practices for perioperative nursing—1992,* Denver, 1992, AORN.

Atkinson LJ: *Berry and Kohn's introduction to operating room technique,* ed 7, St Louis, 1992, Mosby.

Brooks S: *Instrumentation for the operating room,* ed 3, St Louis, 1989, Mosby.

Bryan VS: Troubleshooting arthroscopic equipment, *Orthop Nurs* 9:18, Jan/Feb 1990.

Chapman MW: *Operative orthopedics,* vols 1 and 2, Philadelphia, 1988, JB Lippincott.

Heim A, Pfeiffer KM: *Small fragment set manual,* ed 2, New York, 1982, Springer-Verlag.

Heim A, Pfeiffer KM: *Internal fixation of small fractures,* ed 3, New York, 1988, Springer-Verlag.

Meeker MH, Rothrock JC: *Alexander's care of the patient in surgery,* ed 9, St Louis, 1991, Mosby.

Muller ME and others: *Manual of internal fixation,* ed 3, Berlin, 1991, Springer-Verlag.

Myer V: Restoration of peripheral nerves. In Pho R, editor: *Microsurgical technique in orthopaedics,* London, 1988, Butterworths.

Pho R; General principles of microsurgery. In Pho R, editor: *Microsurgical technique in orthopaedics,* London, 1988, Butterworths.

6

Equipment and Supplies

The nurse who specializes in orthopaedics must possess a mechanical ability for operating many types of equipment and an ability for managing supplies. Organizing and prioritizing activities to provide equipment and supplies for the procedure improves management of orthopaedic patient care.

ASSESSMENT OF NEEDS

Coordination among disciplines is required in order to ensure the availability of equipment and implants for the procedure. The radiology department must be informed of the scheduled procedure if radiography is appropriate. Product representatives must be aware of scheduling and special needs. Suppliers of braces or other equipment should also be notified if such equipment is required. The nurse caring for the patient should communicate with the physician in advance to ensure that necessary implants and special equipment will be available. Nurses with an understanding of the anatomy, orthopaedic procedures, available instruments, and equipment involved provide an outstanding patient care service.

When the patient arrives in the operating room, assessment information should concur with information previously gathered and with the anticipated procedure. The clinical assessment completed in the office assists in preparing perioperative personnel for the implementation of care. Reviewing radiographs or laboratory values validates the plan of care. The assessment ensures that the correct size and type of equipment and supplies are available. Assessment information should be linked to activities such as placement of the tourniquet, positioning of a limb with respect to postural pressure on nerves and blood vessels, and proper placement of diathermy leads.

Preparing the room includes moving equipment and supplies into the room and testing the equipment before the patient's arrival. To prevent injury, proper body mechanics should be practiced when moving equipment. Traffic patterns should be planned to ensure availability of the sterile field to the team members. Reviewing x-ray films and assessing patient information are helpful measures in anticipating placement of equipment. Radiographic units, both portable and fluoroscopy (image intensifier), should be available for use at the beginning of the procedure and draped at the appropriate time.

The expense of equipment and supplies may prohibit multiple purchases; therefore a central storage area is identified if procedures are not consistently scheduled in the same room. Equipment used for orthopaedic procedures should be cleaned following each procedure, before storage. A routine inspection of equipment must be made to ensure safety and function during use. In addition to planning and use, it is necessary to manage a maintenance program ensuring that equipment is routinely checked for proper function.

TYPES OF EQUIPMENT

Radiographic equipment is used for invasive and noninvasive orthopaedic procedures alike. Radiography is used for completion and documentation of the procedure. X-ray equipment and image intensifiers are standard equipment purchased solely for use in the operating room. Three basic views with reference to patient position are used for radiographic examination:

- In *anteroposterior (AP) views* the x-ray tube is placed vertical to the patient's prone or supine body.
- In *lateral views* the x-ray tube is placed horizontal to the patient's prone or supine body.
- In *oblique views* the x-ray tube is tilted at a designated angle to the patient's body.

Portable radiography (x-ray) equipment is used for making AP and lateral x-ray films (Fig. 6-1). It can be anticipated that two x-ray views will be taken at right angles to each other (Fig. 6-2). Fluoroscopy (Fig. 6-3) with image intensification converts an x-ray beam as it passes through the body into an optical image projected onto a television screen. The image can be permanently filmed. An x-ray technician is responsible for operating the radiography equipment, but coordination by the perioperative nurse is vital to ensure availability of the service at the proper time. The x-ray technician requires notification of the time of the procedure in order to prepare equipment and of the type of procedure planned, along with any special positioning that will be necessary. The nurse organizes activities including safety measures, equipment placement, and draping.

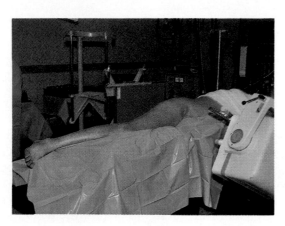

Fig. 6-1 Portable radiography equipment being used preoperatively, before skin preparation.

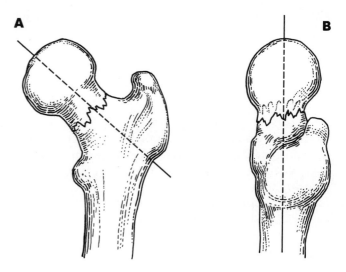

Fig. 6-2 Fracture reduction. **A,** AP view. **B,** Lateral view.

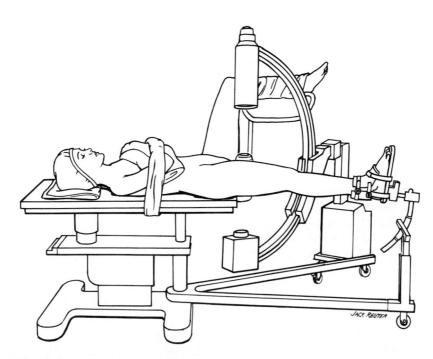

Fig. 6-3 Fluoroscopy (C-arm) equipment positioned after patient has been prepared for procedure.

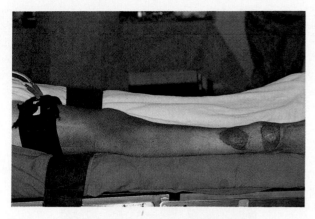

Fig. 6-4   Tourniquet in position before skin preparation.

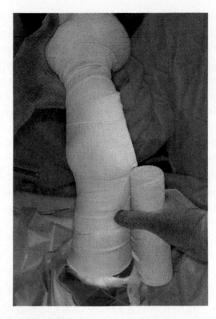

Fig. 6-5   Exsanguination using elastic bandage following elevation of extremity.

Leaded aprons or shields are used to protect the patient and participating personnel. The integrity of leaded shields and aprons should be maintained through preventive monitoring. Radiography badges are used to monitor exposure rates of personnel. Potential radiographic hazards and resulting complications include bone necrosis, cancer, damage to the gonads, and damage to the hematopoietic system. Positioning and draping techniques for the equipment or cassette require implementation of aseptic practices and are completed at the appropriate time depending on the length and type of procedure.

Tourniquets are used to decrease blood supply to the extremity during the surgical procedure, resulting in increased visibility for the surgeon (Fig. 6-4). Tourniquet application and monitoring are required for many orthopaedic procedures, since procedures are commonly performed on an extremity. The pneumatic cuff tourniquet is designed as an automatic pressure-maintaining device that is powered by a cylinder of gas or a battery. The tourniquet should be tested before use, and the gauge should be checked to ensure accuracy. The connectors, cuff, tubing, and ties should be checked for patency and function. Monitoring and maintenance records should be maintained on each tourniquet unit.

Tourniquet application requires assessment of the extremity and location for placement. The site should be assessed to determine whether muscle bulk will protect the underlying nerves. Use of a tourniquet is contraindicated on a limb showing evidence of ischemia from atherosclerosis or at the site of arteriovenous fistula formation.

Tourniquet cuff length and width should be appropriate for the size of the extremity. The tourniquet ends should overlap by at least 3 inches. Recommended cuff lengths are:

Infant arm: 8 inches
Infant leg; child arm: 12 inches
Child leg; small adult arm: 18 inches
Medium adult arm; small adult leg: 24 inches
Medium to large adult leg: 34 inches
Very large adult leg: 42 inches

A wide-cuff tourniquet compresses a greater mass of tissue, resulting in a lower pressure required to provide hemostasis. The cuff may be applied directly to the limb or by using a protective padding placed beneath, such as Webril. Applying the cuff snugly ensures that the expansion will be sufficient to occlude the arteries. Correct sites of application are the thigh (high, close to the groin); the lower leg at the thickest part of the calf; and on the upper arm, a little above the midpoint of the arm, where the muscles are most bulky. Applying a cuff where nerves are superficial and relatively unprotected, such as near a joint, entails the risk of nerve damage and should be avoided. Drawing the skin and subcutaneous tissue distally before placing a tourniquet in obese patients helps to hold the cuff in place. Once the tourniquet is applied, the cuff should not be rotated to a new position or shearing could occur. Placing an impervious drape around the tourniquet prevents pooling of solutions beneath the tourniquet during preparation of the surgical area. The tourniquet should be connected before the patient is draped. A sterile tourniquet may be placed after the patient is draped if tourniquet placement is required close to the incision site. Before the tourniquet is inflated, the limb may be exsanguinated using gravity in combination with an Esmarch (rubber) bandage or an elastic bandage (Fig. 6-5). An Esmarch bandage is applied from the periphery upward with moderate tension to drive the blood in the small vessels proximally. The bandage should be rolled to assist application in a spiral fashion with minimal overlap, extending to the lower edge of the tourniquet cuff. This procedure usually takes place immediately before the cuff is inflated, following draping. Partial exanguination will occur after 2 minutes of elevation, leaving blood in the venous system. Once the cuff is inflated, the Esmarch bandage is removed. The Esmarch bandage should not be used on a limb with an active infection or tumor.

The time of tourniquet inflation is recorded. The pressure setting depends on the patient's age, the systolic blood pressure, the tourniquet width, and the circulation in the limb. Ideally the cuff pressure should be higher than the systolic pressure by 30 to 75 mm Hg in the upper extremity and be one half the systolic pressure in the lower extremity. Maximum duration of tourniquet compression has not been determined, but generally 1 hour for the upper extremity and 1½ hours for the lower extremity have been proved to be safe. Safety depends not on time alone, but also on the pressure of the cuff and the volume of muscle padding. In the early stages of tourniquet compression the danger lies not in ischemia, but in direct pressure on nerves. The higher the tourniquet pressure, the greater the risk of nerve damage. Guidelines for tourniquet placement and tourniquet inflation times are used to make a nursing judgment if the limb is thin or if an unusually high cuff pressure is required because of hypertension. If it becomes necessary to deflate and reinflate the tourniquet during the surgical procedure, blood should be allowed to return to the extremity before the second inflation. The second inflation should be decreased in duration by one half.

Deflation of the tourniquet cuff generally takes place before wound closure to ensure that significant bleeding points are cauterized or ligated to decrease the possibility of hematoma formation. Following removal of the tourniquet cuff, the area is assessed for skin damage or other signs of complications.

Tourniquet use should be documented, including the location of the tourniquet cuff, times of inflation and deflation, tourniquet pressure, and assessment of skin integrity before application and following removal. Tourniquets that are reusable should be cleaned following each use to prevent cross-contamination.

Protective attire is worn in the operating room to protect both patients and personnel. Hoods and bodysuits are available to prevent shedding of bacteria. These filter air breathed by the surgical team and protect team members from being splashed by blood or body fluids. Heavier gloves have been designed for use in orthopaedic procedures to decrease the possi-

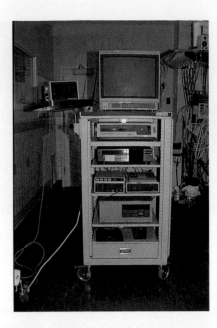

Fig. 6-6 Video system, including monitor, VCR light source, printer, camera, and arthroscopy pump.

bility of penetration by sharp items. Gloves are also available to protect the hands from radiation exposure during procedures requiring x-ray filming or fluoroscopy. In addition, routine attire for all personnel should include masks with shields or other forms of protective eyewear.

Video systems with recorders, monitors, and printers are used for endoscopic and microscopic procedures (Fig. 6-6). A video system allows shared viewing by the assistant at the surgical field and eliminates eyepiece contamination of the sterile field. A videocassette recorder (VCR) allows the surgeon to record all or part of the surgical procedure. The system consists of a small video camera, camera cable, control unit, light source, monitor, and VCR.

Pulsatile lavage pumps (Fig. 6-7) are available for pressure irrigation during a procedure. Antibiotics may be added to the solution. Pulsatile lavage pumps are often used during total joint replacement procedures or for posttraumatic injuries requiring forceful irrigation.

Suction systems with multiple canisters are available for use during procedures requiring large volumes of irrigation solutions, such as arthroscopies. The principle of function is like that of single- or double-vacuum suction, except that use of multiple canisters avoids the need for frequently changing containers.

Positioning devices are used with the standard operating room bed to provide exposure of the surgical site. Patients are positioned for exposure to the op-

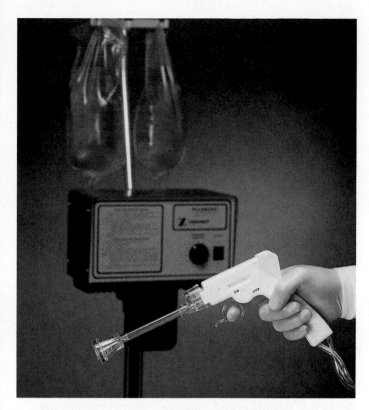

Fig. 6-7 Pulsavac wound debridement system. (Courtesy Zimmer, Inc.)

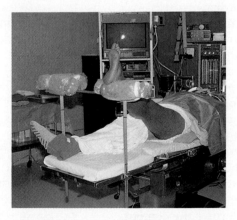

Fig. 6-8 Extremity holder elevating leg for surgical preparation.

erative site in a supine, side-lying (lateral), prone, knee-chest, or other position (see Chapter 4). Accessory attachments are available to be used to support this position. For example, a hand table can be attached to the operating room bed for procedures on the upper extremity. A leg holder (Fig. 6-8) can be attached to the bed for the surgical preparation. This eliminates the need for personnel to hold the extremity.

The leg holder is attached to the bed during procedures on the lower extremity for the purpose of securing the leg in place during the procedure. It is important to assess the pressure caused by gravity on the leg, when positioning it, to prevent nerve damage.

A vacuum pack (Vacpac) can be used to maintain the patient's lateral or semilateral position. Air is removed from the Vacpac by suctioning after the Vacpac is contoured in the desired position.

The three-point positioner is used as a table attachment in three places against the patient's body after the desired position is attained. This is used to support the patient in a lateral position.

The fracture table (see Fig. 6-3) is used for many operations requiring traction, image intensification, or cast application. Use of the fracture table offers the following advantages:

- Fewer assistants are required.
- Manipulation is reduced to a minimum.
- Constant position is maintained.

The table consists of a system of tubular leg supports attached to a small, movable area for resting the patient's torso. Attachments are available to allow any position and traction on any part of the body. Standard component attachments include three-section patient body supports, a lateral body brace, a sacral rest, and traction apparatus. Optional accessories are available to accommodate the need for the types of procedures performed and the style of the table. When the fracture table is to be used, the necessary attachments should be assembled. Parts of the table should be padded with Webril wrap to prevent pressure on joints, the sacrum, and the perineum and to prevent skin breakdown or nerve damage.

Power supplies are operated using compressed air, nitrogen, or batteries to provide power for pneumatic tools and tourniquets. Nitrogen or compressed air may be provided in tanks or through wall outlets. Tanks are equipped with two gauges; one indicates the amount of gas available for use, and the other is for setting the pressure to be delivered. A tank with less than 500 pounds per square inch (psi) should not be used, since this volume rarely provides enough gas to complete a procedure. Pressure settings cannot be verified until the pressure gauge is opened and the power equipment activated. At completion of the procedure, the gas supply should be turned off and the power equipment exhausted of gas from the lines by running the equipment.

Cast material is plaster, fiberglass, thermoplastic, or cast tape of a polyester-cotton blend. Casts provide immobilization to permit healing, to stabilize, to relieve pain, or to assist in realigning tissue. Casts are often applied following a closed reduction by manipulation or following a surgical procedure requiring

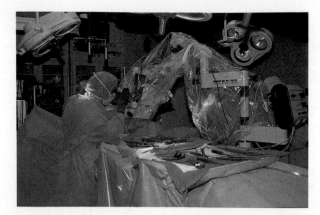

Fig. 6-9 Preparing draped microscope before surgical procedure by checking opticals and visualizing surgical site.

stabilization (see Chapter 8). A cast saw is used for removal of a cast before a surgical procedure is done. Cast removal should be completed in an area other than the operating room that has been prepared for the surgical procedure.

Microscopes and instruments for use during microsurgery procedures are increasing in popularity for orthopaedic procedures. The microscope is draped (Fig. 6-9) at the time of the procedure using an aseptic technique. The principles of microsurgery apply, including care and handling of instruments and equipment. Microsurgery instruments are delicate and should be protected on the field and during cleaning and packaging. The instruments should never be stacked. The microscope should be handled carefully when it is moved and should be protected from jarring during storage. It should be equipped with twin heads with at least one tiltable binocular head for the primary physician. Lenses and oculars should be protected when the drape is removed. The role of the scrub personnel during microsurgery procedures requires constant attention to instrumentation, equipment, and supplies, allowing the surgeon to direct full attention to the field. Microsurgery techniques and instruments vary for orthopaedic procedures because of the many different anatomic structures that are surgically corrected.

Laser use in orthopaedics has been developed into a useful adjunct for arthroscopic procedures for treatment of intraarticular problems, such as abrasion chondroplasty, meniscectomy, and synovectomy, as well as sculpting of articular cartilage and menisci. Lasers are also being used for treatment of herniated disks. For protection of the patient and other personnel, personnel must be certified in laser use in order to operate the laser.

Polymethyl methacrylate (PMMA), an acrylic cementlike substance, has been developed to allow securing of a prosthesis to bone. The idea for a prosthetic grouting agent in total joint replacement was conceived by Charnley, who used pink dental acrylic in the first procedures. The PMMA serves as a buffer for even weight distribution and for other stresses between the implant and the bone. Indications for use of PMMA are to fix prostheses to living bone in procedures for osteoarthritis, rheumatoid arthritis, traumatic arthritis, avascular necrosis, sickle cell anemia, collagen disease, severe joint destruction secondary to trauma or other conditions, and revision of previous arthroplasty procedures. Use is contraindicated in patients with infectious arthritis, active infection of the joint, or joints being replaced when there is a history of infection. It is also not recommended in procedures where the musculature and neuromuscular status are compromised, rendering the procedure unjustified. PMMA is available with radiopaque and nonradiopaque properties.

It is believed that adverse reactions are caused not necessarily by the inserted substance, but by the rise in the intramedullary canal pressure. Monitoring of the blood pressure and pulse is required while the cement is being forced into the canal. Reactions include:

Intraoperative
   Cardiac arrest
   Thromboembolism and/or pulmonary embolism
   Cardiovascular accident
   Sudden death
   Transitory fall in blood pressure
   Hemorrhage and hematoma
Postoperative
   Loosening or displacement of prosthesis
   Surgical wound infection
   Trochanteric bursitis or separation

Methods of preventing a reaction include use of canal cement plugs, venting the cement into the femoral canal, and lavaging the intramedullary canal before inserting the cement.

When the liquid and powder are mixed, a paste is formed. The methyl methacrylate monomer may change in structure over time; therefore the shelf life of the PMMA must be carefully observed. The final cement mass is a composite of powder cemented together by polymerized monomer and entrapped air bubbles. Centrifuging and vacuum mixing reduce porosity and improve fatigue strength. If PMMA is prepared manually, rapid forceful mixing should not be done. The cement hardens in 10 to 12 minutes, but times vary with the batch, manufacturer, temperature and humidity during storage and handling, mixing method, age of the cement components, and thickness

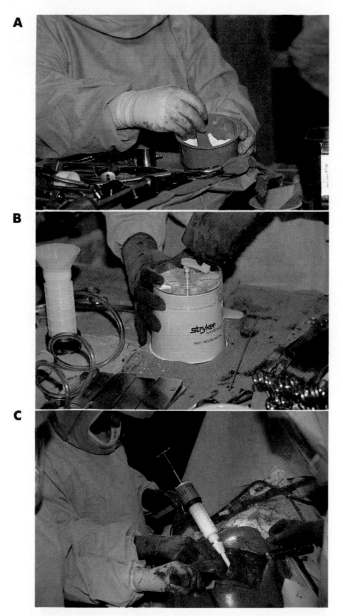

Fig. 6-10 Mixing bone cement, **A**, manually and, **B**, using vacuum system. **C**, Injecting with cement gun.

Products available for use with methyl methacrylate include vacuum systems, centrifuge products, and cement guns (Fig. 6-10).

Wound drainage systems are used to minimize dead space and provide a mechanism for monitoring bleeding or a mechanism for autotransfusion. Orthopaedic surgery frequently leaves large areas of bleeding bone surfaces, requiring closed suction-drainage. To prevent exsanguination, drains are not placed on bleeding bone surfaces or within the intramedullary canal. The drain should be large enough to prevent being plugged by clots. Following placement of the drain in the surgical site, the tubing may be connected to suction until closure is completed. At that time the drainage collection apparatus is engaged and connected. Following closure the drain should be secured with a suture or within the dressing to prevent accidental removal. Autotransfusion systems are available to collect the blood drained from the incision site for postoperative transfusion. Each of these systems has special precautions for use.

Dressings placed on an incision following an orthopaedic procedure will vary according to the preferences, anatomy, and postoperative activities of the patient (Fig. 6-11). Often a soft dressing, including a contact layer of impregnated material such as Adaptic gauze or Xeroform, is applied, followed by an intermediate layer of gauze. Dressings on an extremity are also wrapped with an absorbent dressing, followed by an elastic bandage as a securing layer. Surgical procedures on the knee or shoulder joint may warrant use of a hot ice pack wrapped within the dressing (Fig. 6-12).

Splints and braces are applied following the surgical procedure. Use of these is based on physician preferences, the activity level of the patient, and the need for immobility (Fig. 6-13).

Passive motion devices (Fig. 6-14) are applied in the postanesthesia care unit following some procedures on the knee, elbow, shoulder, and hip. Specific procedures include total knee arthroplasty, supracondylar fractures, tibial plateau fractures, ligament repairs, total hip arthroplasty, hip fractures, postfemoral shaft fracture fixation, total elbow or shoulder arthroplasty rotator cuff repair, and removal of loose bodies. A passive motion device may also be used for the patient who has an infection. The treatment benefits include:

- Inhibited formation of adhesions
- Improved intraarticular cartilage nutrition due to improved fluid mechanics
- Improved clearance of enzymes and exudate from the joint
- Improved matrix formation due to stimulation of chondrocytes

of the cement. Higher room temperature, humidity, and larger cement masses also raise the temperature reached during setting. Temperatures as high as 107° F have been recorded in a block 10 mm thick. Mixing small amounts of antibiotic powder with the cement does not alter its fatigue properties significantly, although liquid antibiotics will markedly weaken the cement.

Pressure injection with a cement gun increases bone penetration of the cement. The prosthesis must be held securely until the position is fixed. Excess cement is removed before the cement is totally hardened.

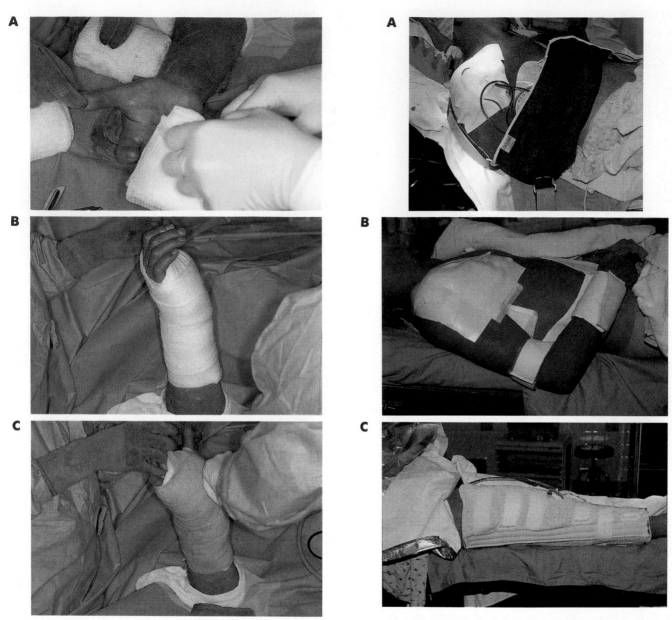

Fig. 6-11 Dressing application. **A,** Contact layer. **B,** Intermediate layer. **C,** Securing layer.

Fig. 6-13 Immobilizer for, **A** and **B,** shoulder (two types) and, **C,** knee.

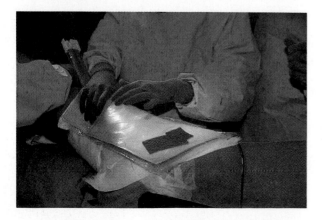

Fig. 6-12 Hot ice incorporated in dressing.

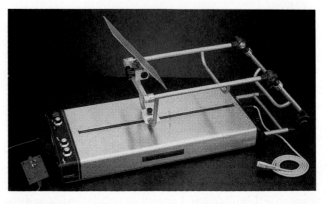

Fig. 6-14 Continuous passive motion device. (Courtesy Stryker Surgical.)

- Early functional range of motion postoperatively
- Decreased postoperative pain, joint stiffness, and swelling
- Decreased recovery time

POSTOPERATIVE COMMUNICATION

The use of multiple types of equipment and variations in supplies requires safety measures during use and postoperative evaluation to ensure that patient care is not compromised. Surgical procedures and physician preferences result in wide variations in care; therefore specific postoperative needs can be met only with communication between caretakers. The intraoperative nurse should document and report information that will assist the person caring for the patient in the postanesthesia care unit (PACU) to evaluate intraoperative care. Neurovascular status, skin integrity, assessment of dressings for drainage or bleeding, patency of drains, and output are a few of the PACU nursing observations. Preoperatively, patients should have been taught what to expect following surgery as a result of the equipment and supplies to be used. If the patient understands the position he or she was placed in during the procedure, it is easier to explain a transient postoperative muscle ache. Patients also should understand the dressings, splints, or other recovery needs associated with the procedure. Documentation of preoperative teaching provides continuity and reinforcement of the patient's discharge instructions.

BIBLIOGRAPHY

Association of Operating Room Nurses: *AORN standards and recommended practices for perioperative nursing—1992*, Denver, 1992, AORN.

Chapman MW: *Operative orthopedics*, vols 1 and 2, Philadelphia, 1988, JB Lippincott.

Meeker M, Rothrock J: Alexander's care of the patient in surgery, ed 9, St Louis, 1991, Mosby.

PART TWO

Surgical Interventions

7

Acquired Musculoskeletal Disorders

Acquired musculoskeletal disorders occur with metabolic changes, degenerative changes, structural changes, or tumor formation. Surgical intervention can correct a skeletal problem but does not always change the disease process. Osteoporosis and arthritis are two of the most common degenerative disorders. Surgical intervention is not always indicated for these disorders unless pain or limited range of motion results in a change in lifestyle. Other acquired disorders include formation of ganglia, development of synovitis, or neurologic changes. Tumors may arise as primary growths or spread secondarily to the bone from another location. Each type of tumor requires individualized intervention, since not all tumors can be surgically treated. Patients with acquired musculoskeletal disorders requiring surgical intervention may be in any age group.

NURSING CARE

Nursing diagnosis will vary depending on the musculoskeletal disorder being treated and the patient's age, medical history, and surgical history, as well as other factors. Nursing care for the patient undergoing surgical procedures to correct a musculoskeletal problem is consistent with that provided for other patients (see Chapter 4). Priority nursing diagnoses, preoperative planning, and interventions for a patient with an orthopaedic disorder may include:

Priority Nursing Diagnoses	Preoperative Planning and Interventions
Altered tissue perfusion related to: Type of procedure Medical history, including vascular integrity Use of tourniquet	Assess and document: Peripheral pulses Extremity warmth Capillary refill Apply pneumatic tourniquet correctly, verify pressure settings, monitor throughout the procedure, and assess
Anxiety and/or fear related to: Knowledge deficit regarding planned surgical intervention and outcome Immediate discharge home	Provide explanations and reassurance to the patient and family Reinforce patient teaching and answer questions as needed Review discharge plans and instructions; encourage participation in discharge planning Verify understanding of signs and symptoms to be reported Provide information to the family or signficant other during the procedure
Pain related to: Current medical status and degree of involvement	Provide adequate assistance when moving, during transfer Provide explanations Assess and maintain comfort by positioning

Priority Nursing Diagnoses	Preoperative Planning and Interventions
High risk for infection related to: Implanted foreign object	Plan the location of the procedure considering the surgical site and equipment to be used so as to maintain traffic patterns in the operating room Monitor sterility of instruments, implants Administer antibiotics per order

Perioperative nursing practices require continual evaluation and revision of the nursing care plan as care is being provided. The plan of care is implemented, and a postoperative assessment is completed. Many interventions cannot be assessed immediately to determine the long-term outcome; postoperative assessment provides baseline information for evaluating the nursing interventions. Priority postoperative assessment data to gather when caring for a patient with an acquired musculoskeletal disorder include readiness for discharge, understanding of instructions for medication therapy, awareness of postoperative physician appointments, signs and symptoms to be reported, and need for and commitment to physical therapy.

Documentation of the care provided and the results of evaluation is completed to provide for continuity of care and a record of that care. Documentation on an intraoperative record is individualized for each setting. A summary of the nursing activities impacting the outcome should be reported to postanesthesia care unit personnel. Information that should be documented and communicated following an orthopaedic procedure varies with the many types of procedures completed for musculoskeletal disorders. The report that is necessary may change in an outpatient versus an inpatient setting, based on the amount of teaching acquired preoperatively and the services available to the patient. Priority information may include:

- Implanted devices as appropriate
- Patency of drains; dressings (drainage, bleeding; intactness)
- Precautions required for positioning
- Fluid loss and replacement
- Preoperative teaching and level of comprehension
- Individualized care provided

The text and photographs in this chapter identify techniques implemented during orthopaedic procedures for patients with musculoskeletal disorders commonly treated as an elective procedure. The procedures depict common surgical approaches and select instrumentation. The procedures do not identify each step of the procedure requiring physician consideration but are intended to provide an overview of the procedure to enable the perioperative nurse to anticipate patient care needs. These procedures can also be implemented for traumatic injuries in the event that a similar course of treatment is considered. Instrumentation, equipment, and physician preference change in each setting; therefore it is important to recognize the principles of each procedure and to consider implementation based on an understanding of orthopaedics as a specialty.

ARTHROSCOPIC PROCEDURES

Arthroscopic procedures involve visualization of a joint through an arthroscope for purposes of diagnosis or treatment; as a result, the pain commonly associated with an open procedure may be minimized and rehabilitation simplified.

Arthroscopy may be performed as a diagnostic procedure or for operative treatment:

Diagnostic: For patients whose diagnosis cannot be determined by the history, physical examination, or arthrogram or when findings are insufficient to warrant surgical exploration. The procedure may be performed before an anticipated operative arthroscopy or arthrotomy for confirmation of findings.

Operative: For patients with an abnormality or injury requiring surgical intervention.

Equipment and Instrumentation Specific for Arthroscopy

Arthroscope—30-degree angle most common

Arthroscopy instrumentation (Fig. 7-1)

Fluid control system (as indicated)

Video equipment, including monitor, printer, and videocassette recorder (VCR)

Camera and light cord

Irrigating solution of Ringer's lactate or normal saline

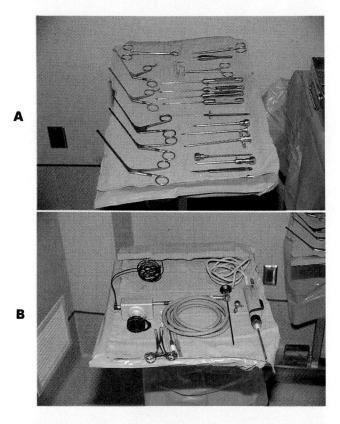

A

B

Fig. 7-1 Mayo trays prepared for arthroscopy. **A,** Arthroscopic instrumentation. **B,** Arthroscope, camera, light cord, and shaver.

Diagnostic or operative knee arthroscopy

DESCRIPTION ■ Direct and thorough examination of the knee joint through the arthroscope. Tiny portals are made, and the joint is inflated. A diagnosis can usually be made at this time. Surgical treatment of meniscus injuries, ligament injuries, wear-and-tear problems, and patella problems can take place through the arthroscope.

INDICATIONS ■ Synovitis, plical adhesions, loose bodies, chondromalacia, osteophytes, degenerative meniscal tears, intraarticular abnormality, or ligamentous injury.

EQUIPMENT AND INSTRUMENTATION ■

See Equipment and Instrumentation Specific for Arthroscopy

Soft tissue instruments

PROCEDURE ■

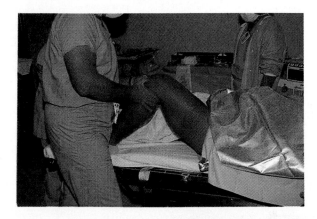

1 An examination with the patient under anesthesia may be completed by the surgeon before the patient is positioned.

2 Equipment is positioned in the room to facilitate viewing the video monitor.

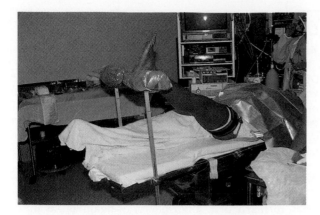

3 The patient is placed in a supine position. The arm on the operative side is padded and taped across the chest. The arm on the unoperative side is left at the side on a padded armboard and secured. The leg holder is positioned to secure the operative leg. A thigh tourniquet cuff is placed on the upper thigh of the affected leg. A heel protector is applied to the heel of the unoperative foot.

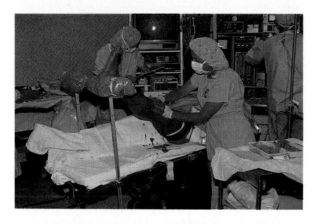

4 The surgical site is prepared beginning with the site of incisions circumferentially. The surgeon's preference may be to prepare the foot.

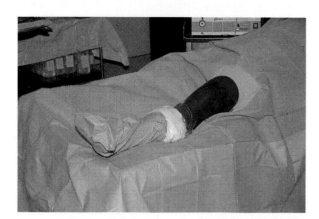

5 The leg is draped free, exposing the surgical site from the tourniquet to midcalf. Equipment and instruments are brought to the operating field.

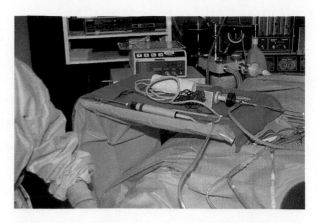

6 The connecting ends of the light cord, shaver, camera, and irrigating tubes are passed off the field to be connected to the source.

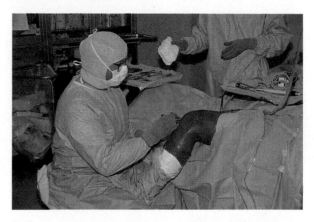

7 The surgical team is positioned to maintain sterility. The incision for the anterolateral portal is made with a No. 11 blade.

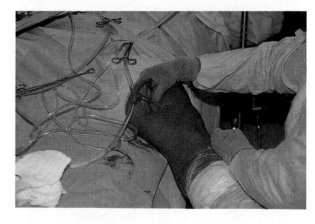

8 The sharp trocar is replaced with the blunt trocar to advance the sheath into the joint.

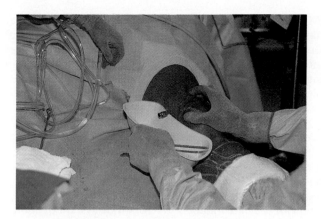

9 The inflow cannula is inserted, and the joint is distended. Irrigation of the joint is performed if necessary.

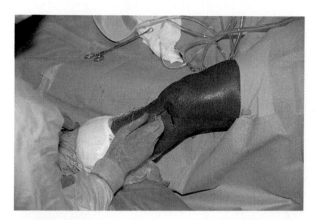

10 The incision for the second portal is made with a No. 11 blade.

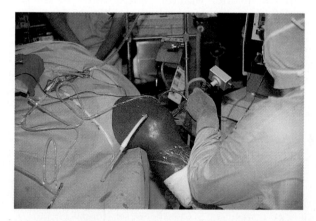

11 The scope sheath and then the arthroscope are inserted. At this time the surgeon inspects the entire joint, including the suprapatellar pouch, the undersurface of the patella, the medial and lateral femoral condyles, the tibial plateaus, and both menisci.

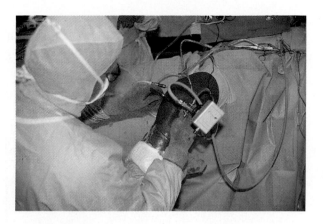

12 A third incision is made for placement of a portal if a pathologic condition is found. Portal placement and instrumentation will depend on the anatomy affected.

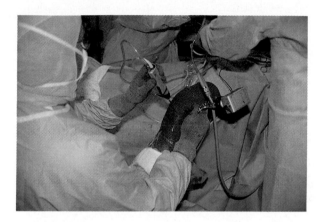

13 Instrumentation is used to remove or correct the pathologic condition.

a Meniscectomy (removal of the meniscus): indicated for a knee that locks or for a torn cartilage that causes recurrent pain and limited movement. Most surgeons prefer to excise the portion that is torn loose. A pseudomeniscus may grow to replace cartilage that has been removed. Leaving the undamaged part also salvages some of the shock-absorbing effect of the normal meniscus.

b Collateral ligament repair: indicated for damage caused by force to the lateral side of the knee while the foot is anchored to the ground. Extreme adduction of the leg is usually necessary to injure the fibular or lateral collateral ligament.

c Chondrectomy (patellar shaving or removal of degenerative cartilage): performed using the arthroscope for shaving the underside of the patella. The end of the femoral condyle may also be shaved. The procedure is indicated for chondromalacia patellae or hypertrophic degenerative changes of the articulating cartilage of the patella that occur following recurrent dislocation or subluxation, repeated minor injury, major trauma, or friction in the femoral groove.

14 The joint is irrigated and deflated. Incisions are closed with a nonabsorbable suture. If absorbable suture is used, Steri-Strips are applied. A dressing and compression wrap is applied.

■ NURSING CARE AND TEACHING CONSIDERATIONS ■

Check equipment for function before each procedure and place it for ease of visualization by the surgical team.

Thoroughly rinse instruments that have been disinfected with glutaraldehyde.

Complete a neurovascular assessment of the extremity.

Provided patient instruction.

Plan for discharge within 4 to 6 hours postoperatively.

Reinforce discharge instructions:

- Ice packs should remain on the incision site for 24 hours.
- Crutch walking with weight bearing can begin within 24 hours.
- Straight-leg exercises are started immediately.

Arthroscopic anterior cruciate ligament reconstruction with patellar tendon substitution

DESCRIPTION ■ Replacement of a torn anterior cruciate ligament with the aid of the arthroscope, using the central third of the patellar tendon with the patellar bone block superiorly and the tibial bone block inferiorly. The placement of this graft must be isometric and in an anatomically appropriate location in order for it to function properly. There are many variables and different guide systems for the procedure. The selection of the guide system is made by the surgeon. The procedure described here uses the Concept Universal Guide System. Anterior cruciate substitution is also made with grafts other than the patellar tendon, such as the semitendinous tendon, the iliotibial band, the gracilis muscle, or the fascia lata. Cadaver tendon has also been used. The ligament can also be strengthened with a ligament augmentation device.

INDICATIONS ■ A torn anterior cruciate ligament that has resulted in simultaneous anterior and rotational stresses. Candidates are usually active, and the injury has interfered with their activities. Failure to respond to bracing, rehabilitation, exercise, or other nonoperative treatment has resulted in the need for operative repair.

EQUIPMENT AND INSTRUMENTATION ■
See Equipment and Instrumentation Specific for Arthroscopy
Positioning equipment for drop-knee position
Soft tissue instruments
Large-bone instruments
Anterior cruciate ligament (ACL) guide system of choice (steps of the procedure will vary with the surgeon's choice of system)
Tourniquet
Power equipment

PROCEDURE ■

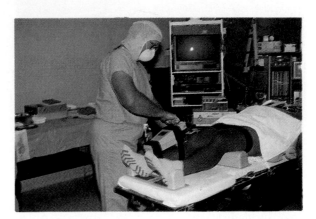

1 An examination with the patient under anesthesia is performed to evaluate the instability of the knee. A KT 1000 examination, a method of applying numbers to the amount of tibial displacement and therefore instability, is sometimes done. The patient is positioned, the surgical site is prepared, and the patient is draped for an arthroscopy. A leg holder may be used to secure the leg throughout the procedure. The arthroscopy is completed.

2 The remaining anterior cruciate ligament tissue is debrided with basket forceps and a powered meniscus resector. A femoral notchplasty is made with a ¼-inch osteotome, a mallet, and a grasper to accommodate the patellar tendon graft.

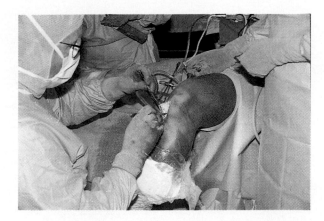

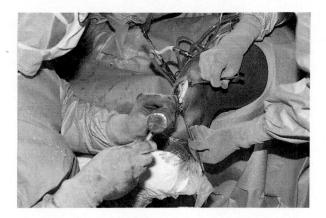

3 The inflow is clamped, and the patellar tendon graft is harvested. An anterior longitudinal incision that parallels the patellar tendon is made with a No. 10 blade, forceps, and retractors. The middle one third of the tendon is used.

6 A ¼-inch curved osteotome and a mallet are used to remove the tibial bone block.

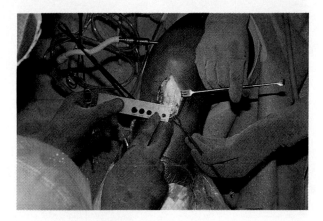

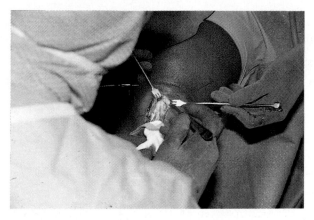

4 The tendon and bone are marked for size.

7 The length of the tendon is dissected using a No. 10 blade and scissors. The procedure is repeated to remove the patellar bone block.

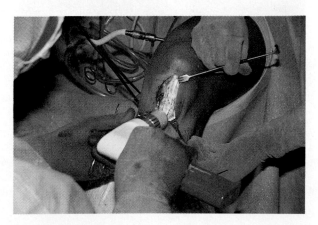

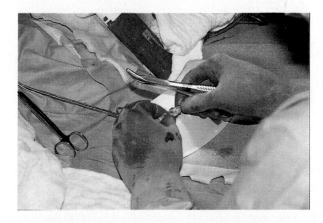

5 A sagittal saw is used to harvest the tibial bone block.

8 Following removal of the graft, a rongeur, scissors, and sizer are used to prepare the bone for insertion. Two or three holes are drilled in the patellar bone and tibia with a ⁵⁄₆₄-inch Steinmann pin or drill bit. Heavy sutures, such as No. 5 Ethibond, are placed in each end of the graft.

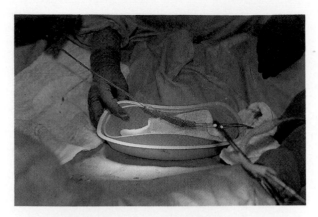

9 The graft is placed in a saline-soaked sponge and secured on the back table.

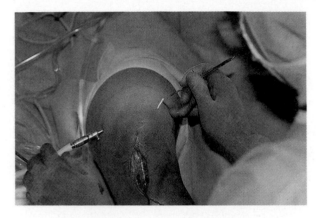

10 A lateral thigh incision is made over the iliotibial band to prepare for femoral drilling.

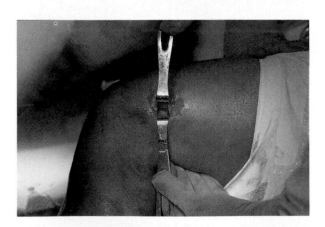

11 The vastus lateralis is retracted, and dissection is completed by the surgeon. A No. 10 blade, forceps, and retractors are used. The joint is cleared of clots of other debris at this time by unclamping the inflow and using the powered meniscus resector.

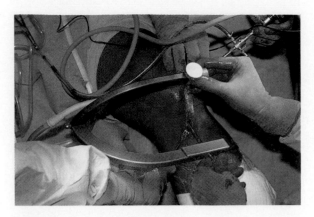

12 The horseshoe guide is placed in the anterior incision.

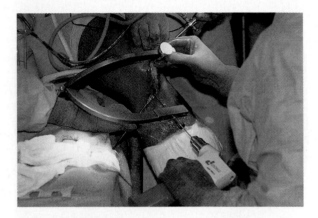

13 The tibial guide pin is placed.

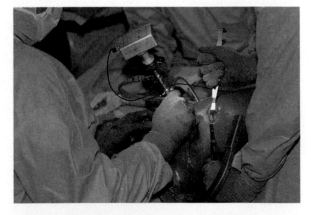

14 The horseshoe guide is repositioned to the lateral incision.

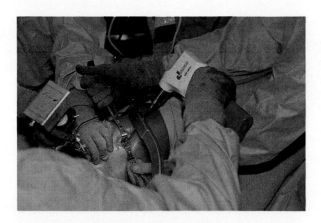

15 The femoral guide pin is inserted.

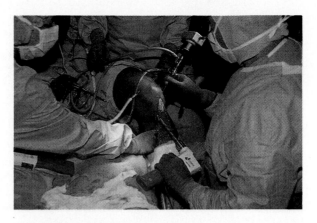

18 The tibial tunnel is drilled with a cannulated reamer.

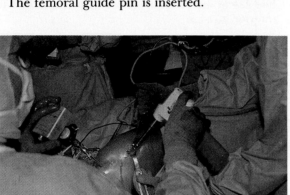

16 The femoral tunnel is drilled with a cannulated reamer.

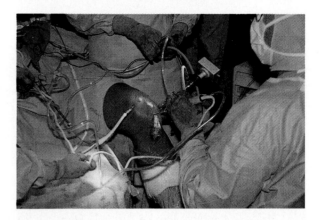

19 The joint is cleared of bone and clots with the powered meniscus cutter.

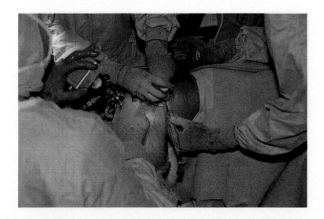

17 A bone plug is placed to maintain joint distension.

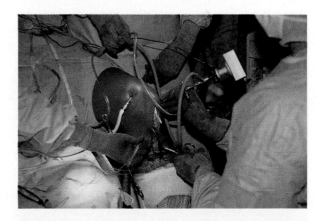

20 The inflow is clamped, and the graft is passed through the joint using a graft passer.

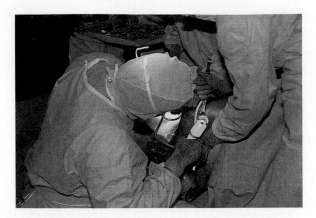

21 The graft is secured superiorly by drilling a hole in the femur with a 3.2 drill bit.

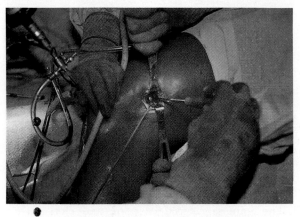

22 A flathead screw is inserted, serving as a post for securing the sutures.

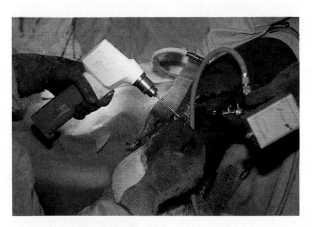

23 The graft is secured inferiorly in the same manner. Isometricity and proper anatomic placement are ensured, and the inflow and arthroscope are removed.

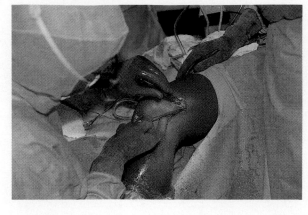

24 The fascia and skin are closed on the lateral and anterior incision.

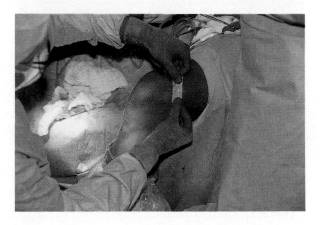

25 The portals are closed with Steri-Strips.

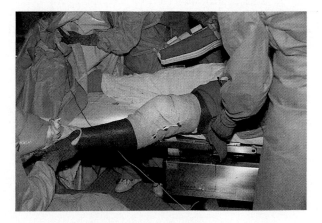

26 A compression dressing is applied.

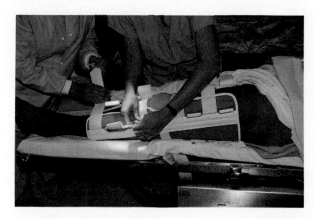

27 A knee immobilizer is applied. A brace may also be used. Hot ice packs can be applied in the dressing.

■ NURSING CARE AND TEACHING CONSIDERATIONS ■

Check equipment for function preoperatively and place it for ease of visualization by the surgical team.

Thoroughly rinse equipment that has been disinfected with glutaraldehyde.

Complete a postoperative assessment of the extremity.

Provide patient instruction:

- Ambulation is started immediately with crutch walking.
- Passive exercise is started immediately; active exercises are started at 10 days to 2 weeks postoperatively.
- Knee immobilization is maintained for up to 4 weeks; activities are gradually resumed over a period of 1 year.

Shoulder arthroscopy

DESCRIPTION ■ Use of the arthroscope to visualize the glenohumeral joint for correction of intraarticular and some extraarticular lesions.

INDICATIONS ■ Chronic shoulder problems, including anterior, posterior, or multidirectional glenoid labrum lesions; biceps tendon and rotator cuff tears; synovitis; loose bodies; instability; adhesive capsulitis; acromial arch decompression; and impingement syndrome. Synovial biopsy, synovectomy, bursectomy, and stabilization of dislocations can be accomplished through the arthroscope.

EQUIPMENT AND INSTRUMENTATION ■

Positioning equipment for the lateral decubitus position with arm suspended

See Equipment and Instrumentation Specific for Arthroscopy

Soft tissue instruments

PROCEDURE ■

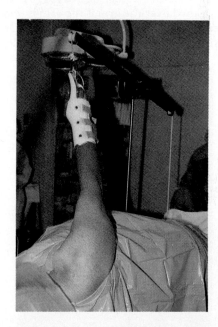

1 The patient is positioned in the lateral decubitus position with the arm suspended on a rope and pulley. Weights are added. Overstretching of the axillary artery is prevented by adding only enough weight to extend the arm.

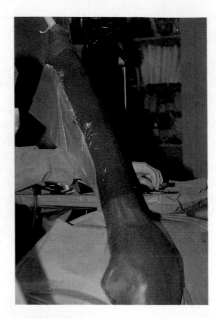

2 The area is prepared from the neck, anterior mid-chest to midscapula, to the waist, including the arm to the elbow. The area is draped by wrapping the arm with a sterile impervious drape. A stockinette can be draped over the arm if the arm is temporarily released from the positioning device. A U drape and split sheet are used to drape the shoulder.

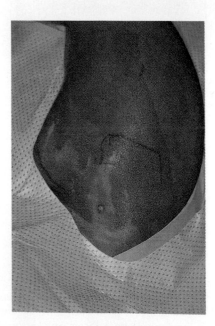

3 The acromion, clavicle, and coracoacromial ligament are marked using a marking pen.

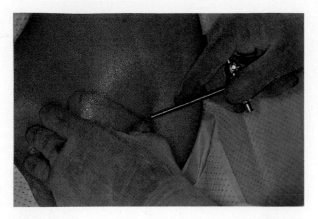

4 Following a stab incision with a No. 11 blade, the arthroscopic sheath with the sharp trocar is introduced in the posterior portal. The sharp trocar is replaced with the blunt trocar to advance the sheath into the joint.

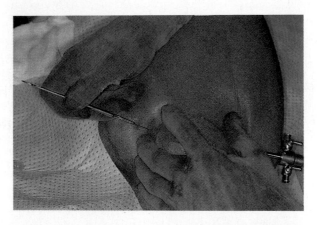

5 A second portal is established with a stab incision using a No. 11 blade.

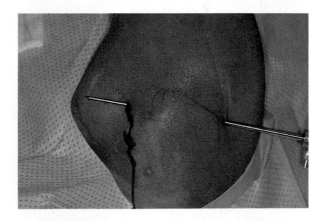

6 A Wisinger rod is used to form the tunnel for the cannula.

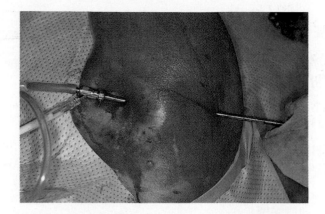

7 The inflow cannula and tubing are connected.

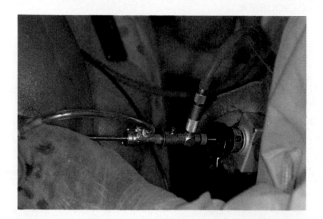

8 The camera and light source are connected.

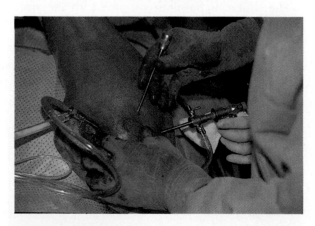

9 A portal is established with a stab incision to use as the port of entry for the operative instrumentation, including the shaver or probe.

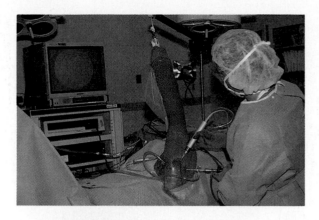

10 Instrumentation is used to correct tears or remove loose bodies while viewing the monitor. The motorized shaver with blades or burs is used for the repair.

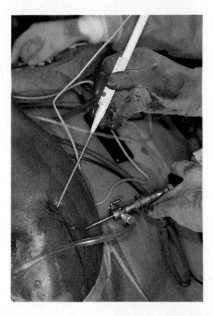

11 An arthroscopic cautery is inserted in the joint for repair. At completion of the procedure the joint is irrigated thoroughly until it is clear of blood and any particles. The portals are closed with a nonabsorbable suture; if an absorbable suture is used, Steri-Strips are applied.

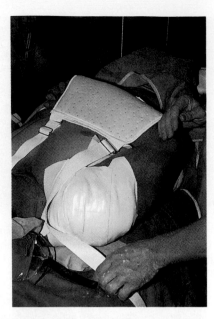

12 A gauze dressing, Webril, and Ace bandages are applied. The extremity is placed in a shoulder immobilizer.

■ NURSING CARE AND TEACHING CONSIDERATIONS ■

Preoperatively, assess range of motion of the extremities to ensure correct positioning.

Postoperatively, assess the neurovascular status of the extremities.

Evaluate the fit of the shoulder immobilizer.

Immobilize the extremity for 24 hours.

Encourage early active motion of the hand and elbow.

Begin gentle-pressure range of motion on the second postoperative day.

Provide active assisted elevation for 3 to 4 days postoperatively.

Endoscopic carpal tunnel release

DESCRIPTION ■ Release of the transverse carpal ligament of the wrist using the endoscopic method.

INDICATIONS ■ Symptoms of carpal tunnel compression; need for decompression of the carpal canal.

EQUIPMENT AND INSTRUMENTATION ■
See Equipment and Instrumentation Specific for Arthroscopy
Soft tissue instruments
Tourniquet
Hand table

PROCEDURE ■

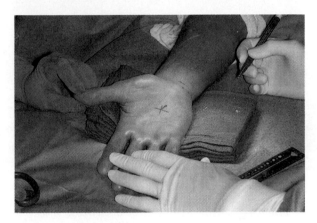

1 The patient is positioned supine with the arm extended on the armboard. A tourniquet is applied on the upper arm. The arm is exsanguinated using an Esmarch bandage, and the tourniquet is inflated. A skin marker is used to identify the entry and exit portals of the endoscopic cannula. The hand is placed on towels for skin incisions.

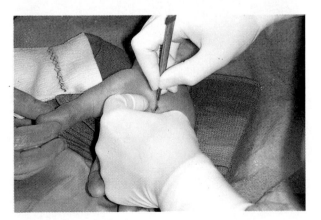

2 A puncture is made in the entry and exit portals using a No. 11 or 15 blade.

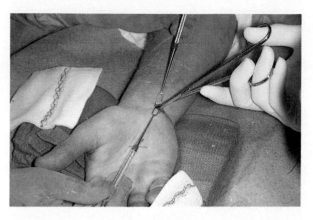

3 The entry portal is dissected using tenotomy scissors.

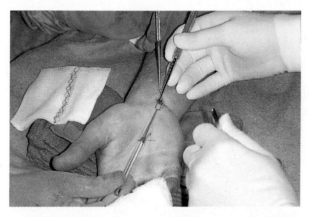

4 A passage is formed using a blunt dissector connecting the entry and exit portals.

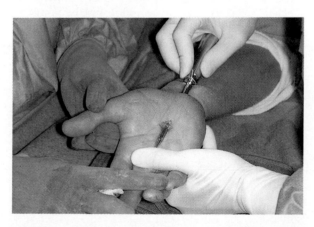

5 The slotted cannula and obturator are passed from the proximal entry portal to the distal exit portal in the palm.

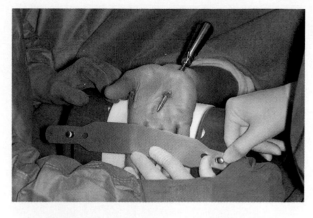

6 The hand is positioned on the hand holder.

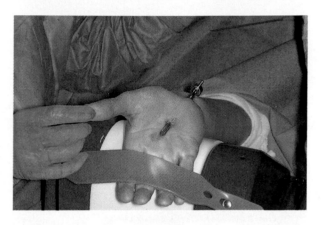

7 The obturator is removed.

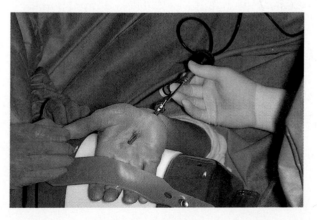

8 The video endoscope is inserted into the slotted cannula.

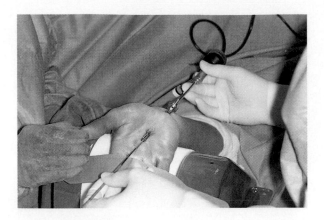

9 The carpal ligament is visualized and explored with a blunt probe.

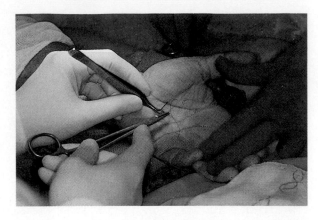

11 The cannula is removed. Each entry portal is sutured with two nonabsorbable sutures.

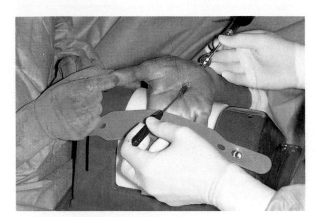

10 The ligament is incised using a series of endoscopic knives through the proximal and distal portals.

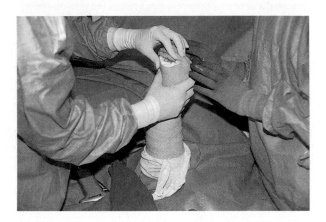

12 A soft dressing is applied using a contact layer on the incision sites, gauze, and Kerlix followed by an elastic wrap. A volar wrist splint may be applied for 2 to 3 days.

■ **NURSING CARE AND TEACHING CONSIDERATIONS** ■

Dressings are removed on the fourth postoperative day.
The splint is removed after 2 weeks.
Full finger range of motion is allowed; wrist motion is limited for 2 weeks.

Ankle arthroscopy

DESCRIPTION ■ Direct examination of the ankle using the arthroscope for diagnostic purposes and for excision, reconstruction, or tissue retrieval for relief of the condition.

INDICATIONS ■ Soft tissue lesions, chondral and osteochondral lesions, or arthritic conditions.

EQUIPMENT AND INSTRUMENTATION ■
See Equipment and Instrumentation Specific for Arthroscopic Procedures
Soft tissue instruments
Tourniquet

PROCEDURE ■

1 Following placement of a tourniquet on the thigh, the ankle is prepared from the toes to the midcalf circumferentially. The foot is draped free using a U drape and an extremity sheet.

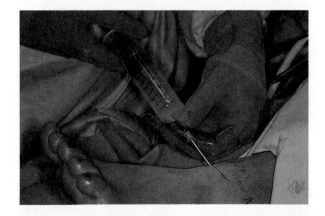

2 The anteromedial aspect of the joint is injected with normal saline using an 18-gauge needle and syringe.

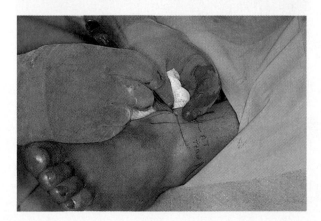

3 A skin incision is made.

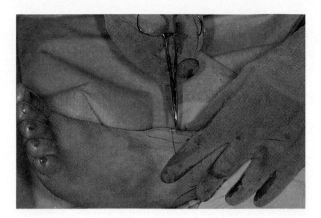

4 Using a small hemostat, blunt dissection is carried out to the level of the capsule.

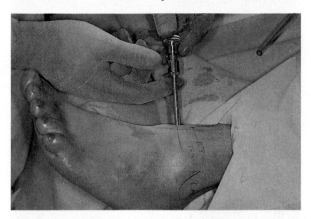

5 The blunt trocar and cannula are inserted in the joint with the foot in a dorsiflexed position.

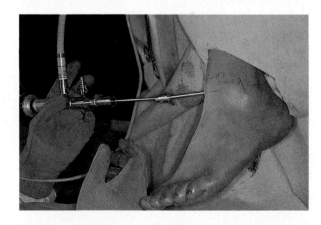

6 The arthroscope is inserted.

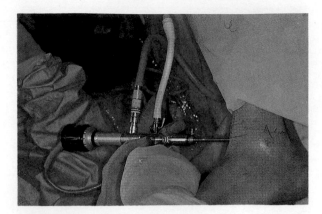

7 The inflow cannula is connected, establishing the anteromedial portal.

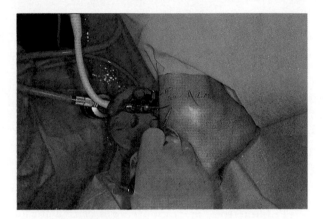

8 A second incision is made over the anterolateral aspect of the joint using transillumination to visualize the incision site and to avoid cutaneous nerves and vessels.

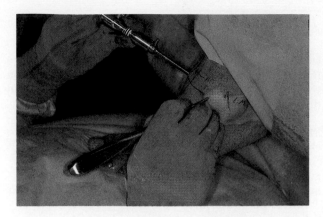

9 Instrumentation is used to treat the problem. Instruments may include:
a Curette

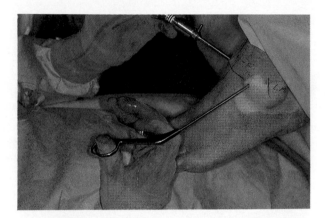

b Grasping forceps

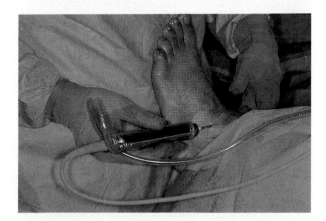

c Shaver

10 The incision site is approximated using a fine, non-absorbable suture.

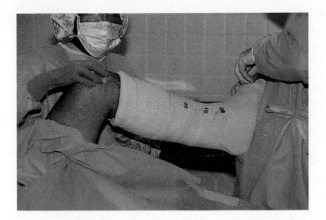

11 A dressing, sugartong splint, and elastic bandage are applied.

■ NURSING CARE AND TEACHING CONSIDERATIONS ■

Check equipment for function preoperatively and place it for ease of visualization by the surgical team.

Thoroughly rinse equipment that has been disinfected with glutaraldehyde.

Provide discharge teaching:
- The extremity should be elevated for 2 to 4 days with cold application.
- Dressings are removed at 3 to 5 days postoperatively.
- Crutches are used for 2 to 6 weeks to maintain non-weight-bearing ambulation.

Begin active range of motion, including progressive resistance exercises with isometrics, 3 to 5 days postoperatively.

SOFT TISSUE PROCEDURES

Soft tissue procedures are used to correct anatomy other than bone. The soft tissues being supported by the bones may be injured by trauma or by "normal wear and tear," or correction of congenital lesions may be necessary. The procedure may or may not require bony involvement. These procedures include repair of such structures as ligaments or musculotendinous units.

Neuroma resection

DESCRIPTION ■ Repair of neuroma (collection of Schwann cells, axon sprouts, and fibrous tissue) by burying the resected neuroma beneath the subcutaneous tissue.

INDICATIONS ■ Painful neuromas resulting from nerve laceration or other injury.

EQUIPMENT AND INSTRUMENTATION ■
Soft tissue instruments
Tourniquet
Hand table

PROCEDURE ■

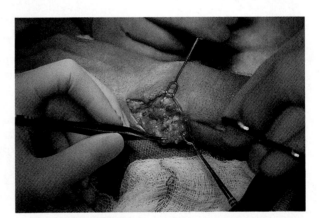

1 The patient is positioned supine with the arm abducted on an armboard. A tourniquet is applied on the upper arm, and the skin is prepared from the fingertips to the tourniquet. The skin incision is marked with a surgical marker. The skin incision is made with a No. 15 blade over the nerve site.

2 Subcutaneous tissue is dissected with tenotomy scissors to the level of the painful nerve ending.

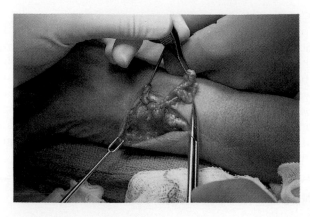

3 Scar tissue is dissected from bulbous nerve endings using scissors (or a Beaver blade).

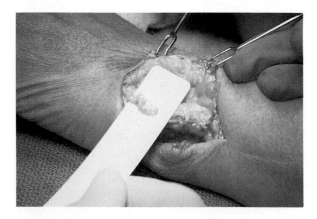

4 Nerve endings are resected sharply and allowed to retract or are buried beneath muscle or padded subcutaneous tissue.

5 Subcutaneous tissue is closed with an absorbable suture, followed by skin closure with a nonabsorbable interrupted or a subcuticular running suture. A soft wrap dressing is applied.

■ NURSING CARE AND TEACHING CONSIDERATIONS ■

Dressings are removed at 10 days postoperatively. Full range of motion is resumed following dressing removal.

Trigger finger/thumb release

DESCRIPTION ■ Release of the first pulley, allowing the tendon to slide and glide easily when the finger is flexed and extended. (Stenosing tenosynovitis, or swelling of the flexor tendon sheath at the level of the first pulley [at the metacarpophalangeal, or MP, joint level], causes the tendon to become caught or stuck as it passes through the narrow pulley when the finger is flexed. The finger/thumb may snap or trigger because the flexor tendons have difficulty sliding through the pulley.)

INDICATIONS ■ Unresponsiveness to nonsurgical management.

EQUIPMENT AND INSTRUMENTATION ■
Soft tissue instruments
Tourniquet
Hand table

PROCEDURE ■

1 The patient is positioned supine, and the hand is extended on the hand table. A tourniquet is applied, the surgical area is prepared from the fingertips to the tourniquet, and the hand is draped free. The hand is exsanguinated, and the tourniquet is inflated.

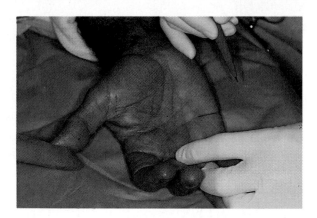

2 The skin is marked for incision in the palm of the hand at the base of the affected finger, distal to the palmar crease for the trigger finger.

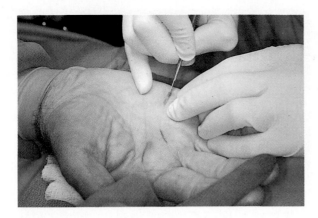

3 An incision is made with a No. 15 blade.

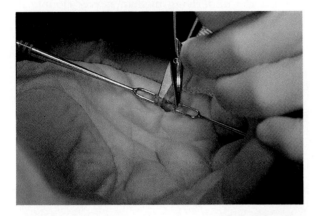

4 Tissue is dissected to the flexor tendon sheath with tenotomy scissors. Double skin hooks are used for retraction. Ragnall retractors may also be used.

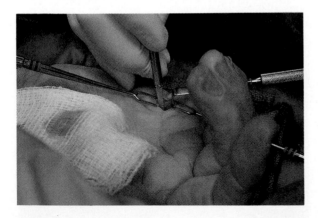

5 A Beaver blade (or tenotomy scissors) is used to dissect the tendon sheath and A1 pulley.

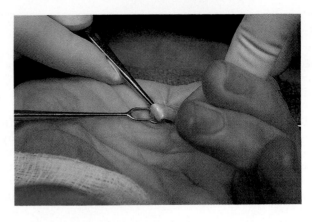

6 The tendon is retracted using a special tendon hook to ensure complete release of the A1 pulley.

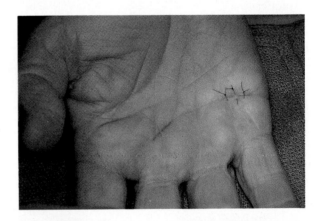

7 Skin edges are approximated with subcutaneous tissue using a nonabsorbable suture.

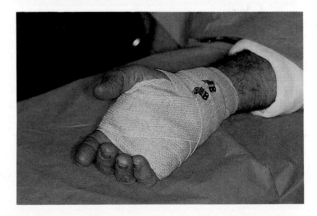

8 A soft dressing is applied and secured with an elastic bandage.

■ NURSING CARE AND TEACHING CONSIDERATIONS ■

The dressing can be removed after 1 week; sutures are removed after approximately 10 days.
Routine hand function is maintained; there should be no heavy lifting or pushing.

Carpal tunnel release

DESCRIPTION ■ Release of the transverse carpal ligament to relieve pressure on the median nerve passing through the carpal tunnel.

INDICATIONS ■ Compression of the median nerve with symptoms of numbness, weakness, or pain caused by edema, bony deformity, or thickening of the tendon sheaths or ligament. Numbness, tingling, and pain are frequently worse at night and may radiate up the forearm. This occurs more commonly in women and may be bilateral.

EQUIPMENT AND INSTRUMENTATION ■
Soft tissue instruments
Tourniquet
Hand table

PROCEDURE ■

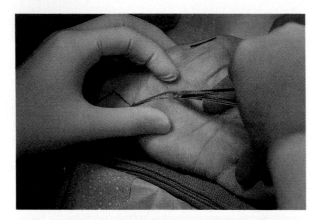

1 The patient is positioned supine with the arm abducted on an armboard. A tourniquet is applied, and skin preparation is completed from the fingertips to the tourniquet. The hand is draped, and the tourniquet is inflated. The skin is marked longitudinally with the skin marker over the ulnar aspect of the thenar crease. The skin is incised with a No. 15 blade; tenotomy scissors are used to dissect through the subcutaneous tissue to the transverse carpal ligament.

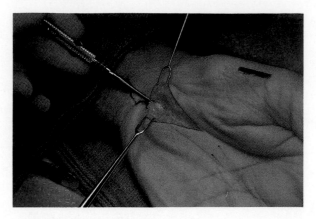

2 A Freer elevator is introduced beneath the edge of the transverse carpal ligament. The Freer elevator protects the underlying median nerve. Double skin hooks are used to retract the skin edges. The transverse carpal ligament is divided using a Beaver blade or tenotomy scissors (not shown).

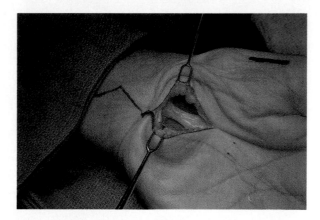

3 The median nerve may possess an hourglass configuration because of compression.

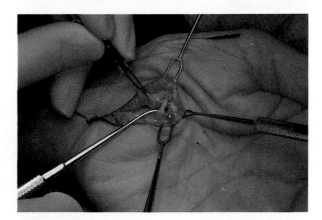

4 The motor branch is inspected using a ball-ended dissector and Bishop forceps. Internal neurolysis of the nerve may be performed using microdissecting instruments. A synovectomy of the flexor tendons may also be performed.

5 The subcutaneous tissue is closed with an absorbable suture. The skin is closed with a subcuticular or interrupted nonabsorbable suture.

6 A soft dressing and plaster splint are applied. An elastic bandage is used to secure the splint. The arm is elevated postoperatively.

■ NURSING CARE AND TEACHING CONSIDERATIONS ■

Assess each finger for color, motion, temperature, and sensitivity.

Provide patient instruction:
- The postoperative dressing is removed after 2 weeks.
- A splint is used for 4 to 6 weeks following dressing removal.
- Wrist range of motion is restricted for 2 weeks; then motion is gradually resumed.
- The dependent position should be avoided.
- Pain associated with carpal tunnel compression is generally relieved following carpal tunnel release. Numbness will be relieved gradually over an undetermined period of time.

Bursectomy of the olecranon

DESCRIPTION ■ Excision of the olecranon bursa, an enclosed sac found between muscles, tendons, and bony prominences. Bursae that are commonly inflamed are the subdeltoid and subacromial bursae of the shoulder; the greater trochanteric bursa; the anserine bursae located between the tendons of the sartorius, gracilis, and semitendinous muscles and the tibia; and the olecranon bursa.

INDICATIONS ■ Recurrent infection or inflammation that cannot be treated with antibiotics or other measures; friction causing edema and inflammation; or tender, painful joint movement.

EQUIPMENT AND INSTRUMENTATION ■
Soft tissue instruments
Large-bone instruments
Power equipment

PROCEDURE ■

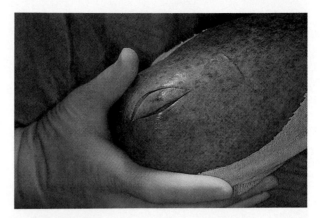

1 The patient is positioned supine with the elbow exposed. The area of excision over the tip of the olecranon is marked.

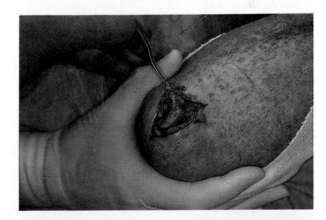

2 An incision is made, and soft tissue is dissected using tenotomy scissors and Adson forceps.

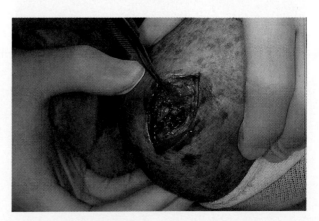

3 The bursal sac is identified and removed, and the tip of the olecranon is exposed.

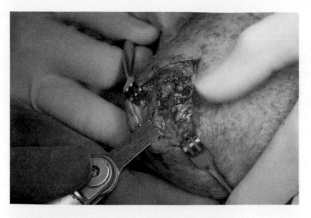

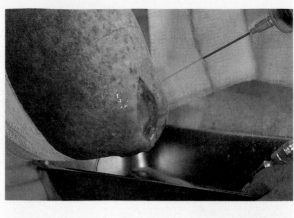

4 The tip of the olecranon is removed:
a Using the power saw with an oscillating blade or

6 The surgical site is irrigated copiously with antibiotic solution.

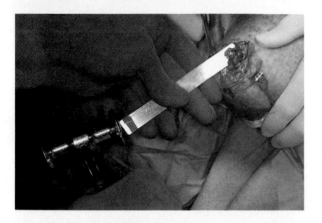

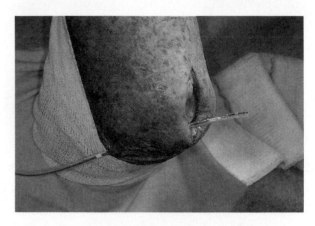

b Using an osteotome and mallet

7 A drain is inserted through a puncture site.

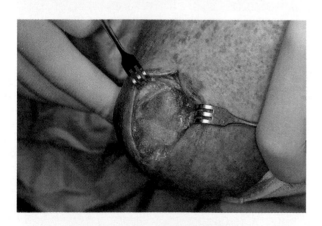

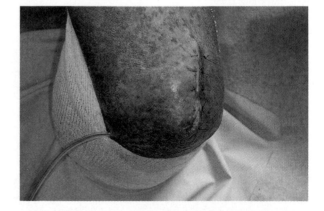

5 The olecranon is removed; bone edges are smoothed (not shown) using a rongeur.

8 The incision site is closed with a subcuticular absorbable suture and nonabsorbable skin suture. A soft compression dressing is applied using a contact layer, gauze, Kerlix, and an elastic bandage. A plaster splint is applied.

■ NURSING CARE AND TEACHING CONSIDERATIONS ■

The drain is removed at 1 day postoperatively.
Dressings are removed at 10 days postoperatively.
Limited range of motion is allowed after 3 to 4 weeks postoperatively.
An elbow pad is used for comfort and protection as long as the patient desires.

SHOULDER REPAIR

Shoulder injuries are caused by trauma, resulting in immediate need for treatment, or most commonly by "wear and tear" on the shoulder joint, resulting in chronic pain and debility. The relationship of the supraspinatus tendon to the shoulder joint, subacromial bursa, coracoacromial ligament, and acromion makes it difficult to diagnose common lesions. Nonsurgical treatment is aimed at symptomatic relief of pain, as well as management of limitation of motion, muscle spasm, and atrophy. Shoulder arthroscopy may be the diagnostic and/or treatment technique of choice for some shoulder lesions. The technique for open surgical correction is determined by the physician; procedures described in this section provide an overview of selected corrective techniques.

Anterior Repair

Capsulorrhaphy for a suspected Bankart lesion

DESCRIPTION ■ A modified Bankart procedure. (The Bankart procedure restores shoulder stability by securing the anterior capsule to bone using holes made in the anterior rim of the glenoid fossa [Fig. 7-2].) In capsulorrhaphy the anterior capsule is overlapped to strengthen the capsule and stabilize the humeral head. Fixation devices are not used for the repair.

INDICATIONS ■ Recurrent anteroinferior glenohumeral instability.

EQUIPMENT AND INSTRUMENTATION ■
Soft tissue instruments
Bankart shoulder instruments
Large-bone instruments

PROCEDURE ■

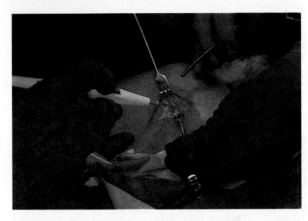

1 The patient is placed in a semisitting position. A small pad may be placed beneath the shoulder. The surgical area is prepared from the chin to the midchest, including the shoulder to the lower arm. The arm is draped free. An anterior axillary incision is made using a No. 10 blade, a cautery for dissection, and Senn retractors for exposure.

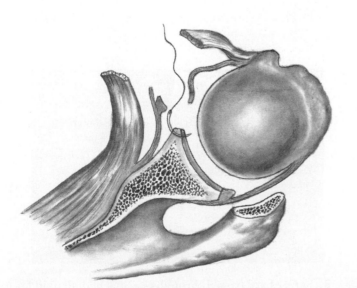
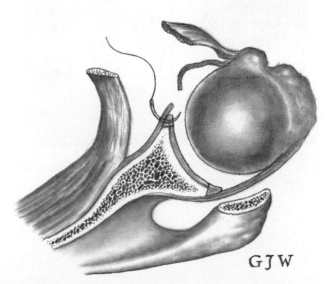

Fig. 7-2 Shoulder repair. Bankart procedure: suture through bone. Capsulorrhaphy: suture through labrum.

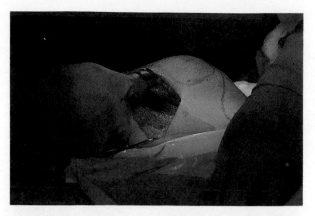

2 Blunt dissection is used to separate the subcutaneous tissue from the deep fascia.

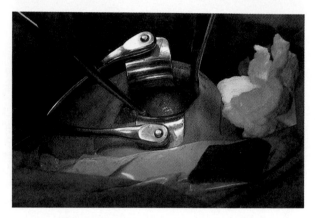

3 A self-retaining retractor is placed to maintain exposure.

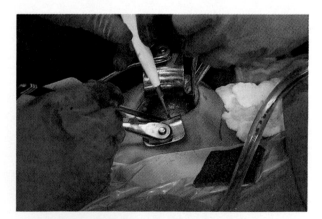

4 The subscapularis tendon is dissected using a cautery. Sharp dissection (scissors) may also be used.

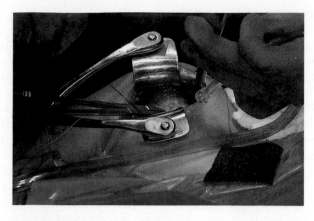

5 Retention sutures are placed using a heavy needle holder.

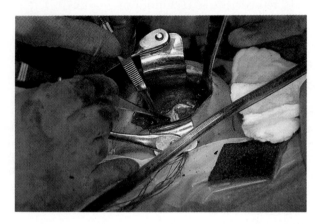

6 The incision is made using a No. 15 blade through the anterior shoulder capsule.

7 The Bankart lesion may be corrected by:
a Using a scaphoid gouge to create holes on the anterior aspect of the glenoid rim and completing them with a curved spike and
b Passing sutures through the glenoid rim and securing the flap

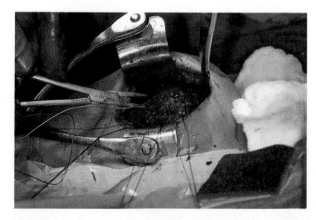

8 Sutures are passed through the attached glenoid labrum.

9 The subscapularis tendon is secured, and the deltopectoral interval is closed using an interrupted absorbable suture.

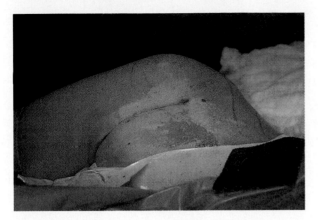

10 Skin closure is completed. Dressings are applied, and a sling or shoulder immobilizer is applied.

■ **NURSING CARE AND TEACHING CONSIDERATIONS** ■

Pendulum exercises are started after 2 days.
Use of the arm is allowed as tolerated.
The sling is used as needed for comfort.
Resistive exercises are started at 3 months postoperatively.
Full range of motion will return in approximately 6 months.

Putti-Platt shoulder repair

DESCRIPTION ■ Reattachment of the lateral portion of the muscle to the anterior rim of the glenoid fossa to limit external rotation.

INDICATIONS ■ Recurrent anterior dislocation of the shoulder.

EQUIPMENT AND INSTRUMENTATION ■
Soft tissue instruments
Large-bone instruments
Bankart instruments
Power equipment
Osteotomes
Curette
Screws

PROCEDURE ■

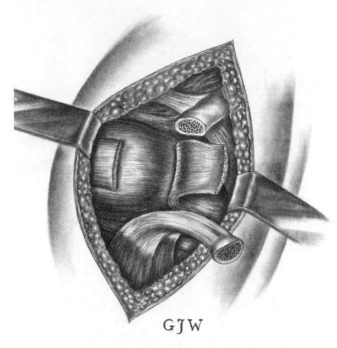

GJW

1 A coracoid osteotomy is performed using an osteotome or a saw. The anterior surface of the subscapularis muscle is exposed. The muscle layer is separated, and stay sutures are inserted.

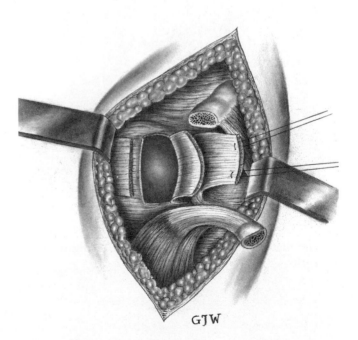

GJW

2 The anterior capsule is opened using a No. 10 blade, and a Bankart retractor is inserted. A curette is used to roughen the scapular neck.

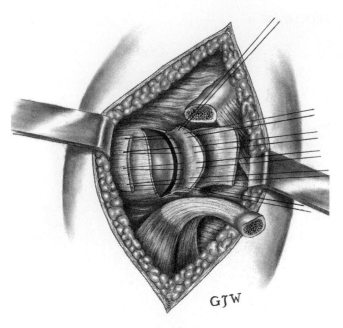

3 Nonabsorbable mattress sutures are inserted.

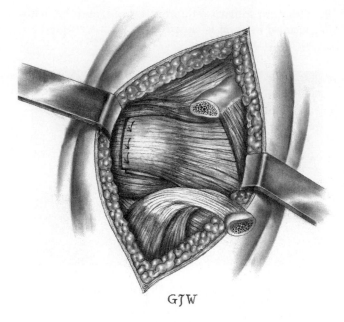

5 The subscapularis layer is secured using mattress sutures.

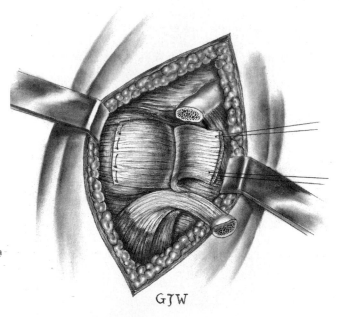

4 The medial capsular layer is secured using mattress sutures.

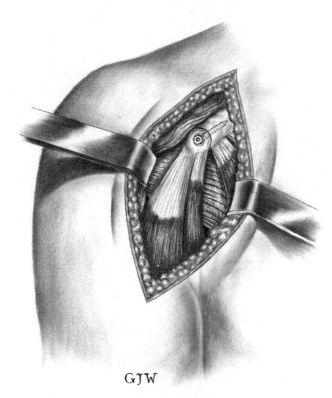

6 The coracoid process is reattached using a 3.5 mm screw.

■ NURSING CARE AND TEACHING CONSIDERATIONS ■

A broad arm sling is applied with the arm secured for 4 weeks; the sling can be worn beneath clothing.

Home exercises are started at 5 weeks postoperatively.

Modified Bristow-Helfet shoulder repair

DESCRIPTION ■ Securing of the coracoid process with the attached tendon of the biceps and coracobrachialis muscle to the glenoid rim.

INDICATIONS ■ Recurrent anterior dislocation of the shoulder.

EQUIPMENT AND INSTRUMENTATION ■
Soft tissue instruments
Large-bone instruments
Power equipment
Screws

PROCEDURE ■

1 Following exposure, a 3.2 mm drill is used to roughen the anteroinferior glenoid rim.

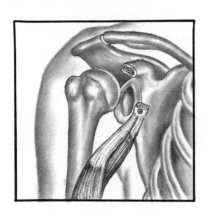

GJW

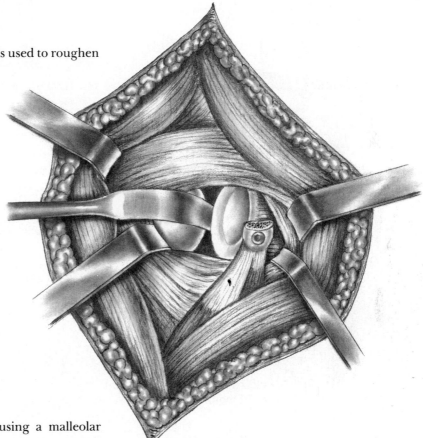

2 The coracoid process is secured using a malleolar screw.

■ NURSING CARE AND TEACHING CONSIDERATIONS ■
Immobilization of the arm is necessary for approximately 8 days. External rotation is limited until the second to third postoperative week.

Magnuson-Stack shoulder repair

DESCRIPTION ■ Reattachment of the subscapularis muscle to the humeral tuberosity for limitation of external rotation.

INDICATIONS ■ Recurrent anterior dislocation of the shoulder.

EQUIPMENT AND INSTRUMENTATION ■
Soft tissue instruments
Large-bone instruments
Osteotomes

PROCEDURE ■

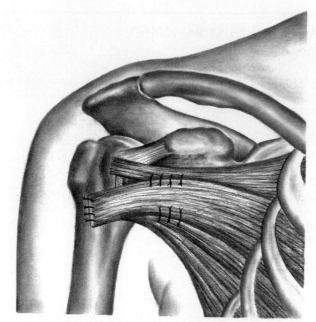

GJW

2 The subscapularis insertion is transplanted to the greater tuberosity and secured with staples or sutures.

> ■ NURSING CARE AND TEACHING CONSIDERATIONS ■
>
> The upper arm is immobilized in a sling for 3 to 6 weeks postoperatively.

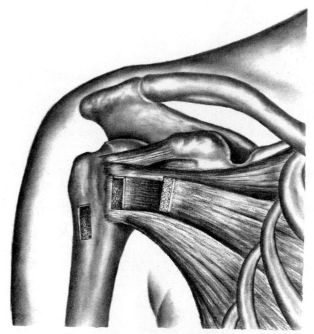

GJW

1 The central portion of the subscapularis muscle is separated, and a small wedge of bone is detached using an osteotome.

Posterior Repair

In a **glenoid osteotomy,** a scapular osteotomy is performed at the level of the glenoid tubercles, and a bone block, taken from the acromion, is inserted.

In a **glenoplasty,** an acromial bone block is screwed to the posterior glenoid border.

The degree of joint separation dictates the degree of treatment. Injuries are commonly caused by (1) horizontal force causing intraarticular damage and (2) downward and laterally rotating force damaging the acromioclavicular (AMC) ligaments. These do not usually require surgical intervention.

Complete dislocation of the AMC joint and disruption of the coracoclavicular ligament cause the clavicle and scapula to separate widely and the shoulder to drop. Methods of repair may include internal fixation that can be removed after approximately 6 weeks to prevent complications.

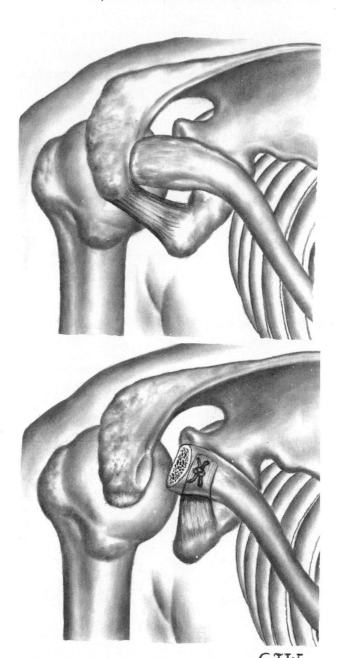

GJW

Weaver-Dunn shoulder repair

DESCRIPTION ■ Insertion of the coracoacromial ligament into the medullary cavity of the clavicle.

INDICATIONS ■ Recurrent dislocation of the shoulder.

EQUIPMENT AND INSTRUMENTATION ■
Soft tissue instruments
Shoulder instrumentation (retractors)
Power equipment

PROCEDURE ■

1 The clavicle is exposed.

2 The lateral end of the clavicle is resected using an oscillating saw.

3 A large drill hole is made in the lateral end of the clavicle. Two drill holes are made in the superior cortex of the clavicle, and the coracoacromial ligament is anchored using a nonabsorbable suture.

■ NURSING CARE AND TEACHING CONSIDERATIONS ■

Immobilization of the arm is necessary for approximately 8 days.
External rotation is limited until the second to third postoperative week.

SPINAL REPAIR

Spinal surgery may require a posterior approach, an anterior approach, a combination posteroanterior approach, or other approaches depending on the anatomy being corrected. Laminectomy is the removal of a vertebral lamina for exposure of the spinal cord and adjacent structures. The terms *laminectomy* and *hemi-laminectomy* are used interchangeably for surgical procedures for correction of herniated nucleus pulposus, spinal cord compression, or fracture. These same conditions may be corrected through the anterior approach.

Anterior cervical discectomy and fusion

DESCRIPTION ■ Removal of the cervical disk and placement of a bone graft for stability.

INDICATIONS ■ Cervical spondylosis, herniated disk, or anterior cervical lesions.

EQUIPMENT AND INSTRUMENTATION ■
Laminectomy instruments
Curettes
Osteotomes
Gouges
Power equipment
Headrest for positioning

PROCEDURE ■

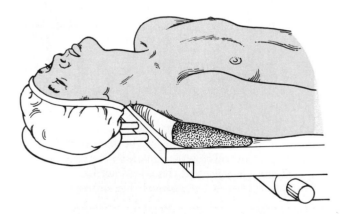

1 The patient is positioned supine in anatomic alignment using a horseshoe headrest. The arms are extended and protected at the sides using Kerlix gauze wrapped around the wrists. The gauze is positioned with the ends hanging free from the end of the operating room bed. Gauze is used to retract the arms if exposure is needed during the procedure.

2 An incision is made, and hemostasis is obtained using a cautery.

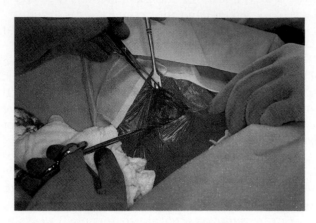

3 Senn rakes are placed for retraction. Tenotomy scissors and Cushing forceps are used for dissecting.

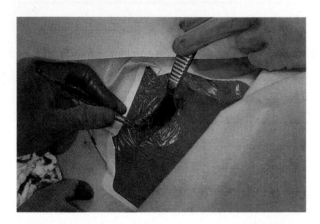

4 A hand-held retractor is used to expose the disk.

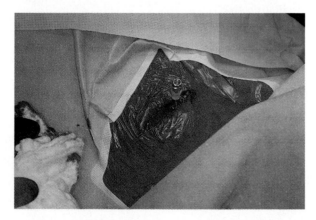

5 A spinal needle is placed in the disk space, and fluoroscopy is used to verify the site.

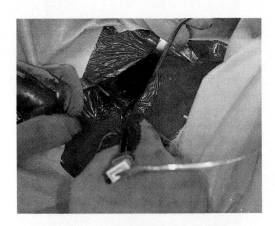

6 A bipolar electrosurgical forceps is used to obtain hemostasis as retraction is maintained for exposure.

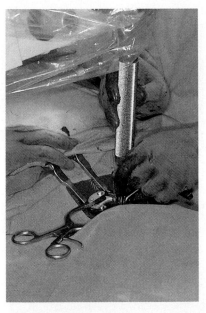

7 A self-retaining retractor is placed below the anterior longus muscle. A Cobb elevator is used to elevate the anterior ligament and muscle from the spine.

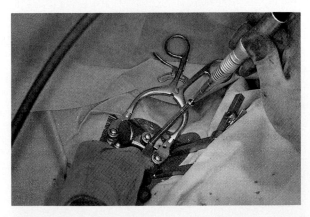

8 A twist drill bit is placed using power as the drill guide provides parallel positioning.

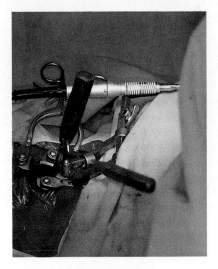

9 A distraction pin is placed above and below the disk space using a screwdriver.

Steps 8 and 9 are repeated on the opposite side to provide exposure with the retractor.

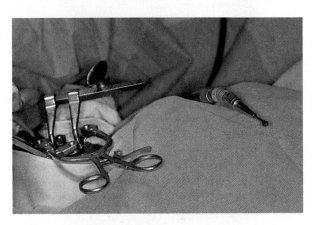

10 A vertebral body distractor is placed bilaterally over the pins, and the body is distracted. Tissue is removed using a pituitary rongeur.

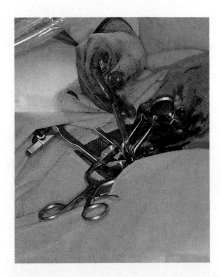

11 A No. 11 blade is used to incise the annulus of the disk.

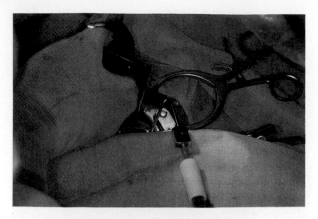

12 The pituitary rongeur is used to remove disk material.

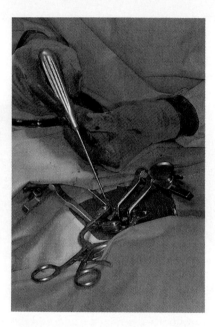

13 A small curette is used to remove disk material, cartilaginous material, and osteophytes.

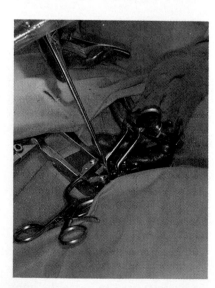

14 A 1 mm Kerrison rongeur is used to remove disk material.

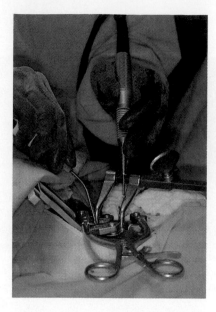

15 A small burr is used to prepare the end plate of the vertebra for the graft.

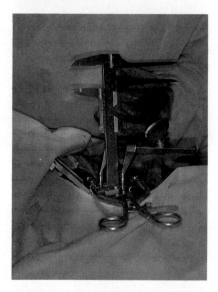

16 A caliper is used to measure disk space for the bone graft.

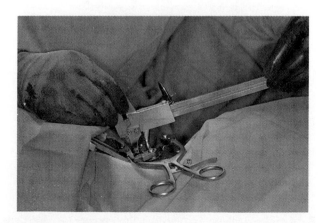

17 The graft site is measured.

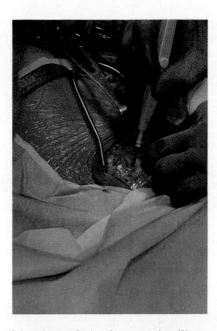

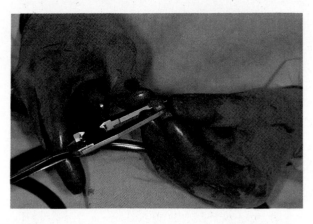

21 The size of the bone block is measured with a caliper.

18 An incision is made in the anterior iliac crest with a No. 10 blade. Tenotomy scissors and a cautery are used to dissect to the crest. Weitlaner and Army-Navy retractors are used to obtain exposure. (Not shown: the crest is exposed using a Cobb elevator.)

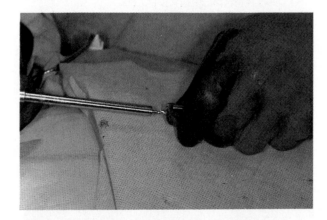

22 A drill bit is placed in the bone block.

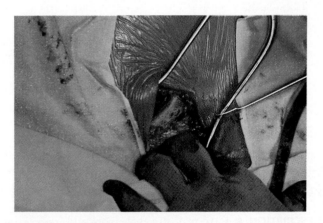

19 The iliac crest is exposed.

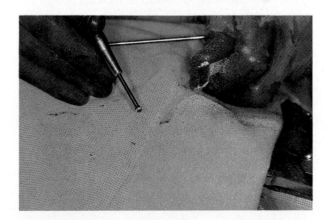

23 The round bur is used to remove excess bone from the block to ensure that the correct size is attained.

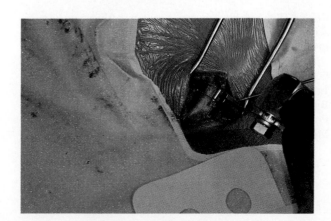

20 A bone block is excised with a double blade on the power saw. The incision site is closed.

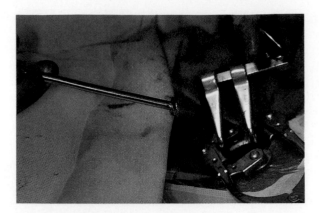

24 The bone block is placed in the cervical space using a drill bit to hold the bone. The drill bit is removed.

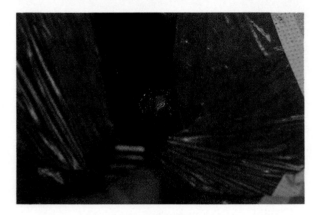

25 The cervical bone is replaced with the bone block for fusion.

26 Subcutaneous tissue is approximated using an absorbable suture.

27 The skin is approximated using an absorbable subcuticular stitch.

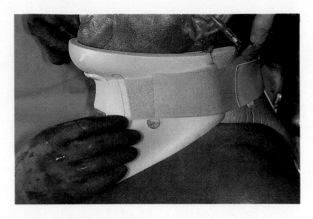

28 The dressing is applied; a neck brace, measured to fit the patient, is applied.

■ NURSING CARE AND TEACHING CONSIDERATIONS ■

Immediately postoperatively, airway management is a priority. The head of the bed remains elevated.
Ambulation is started immediately.
The patient can expect to be discharged within 4 to 72 hours.
The neck collar is worn for 6 weeks.
Isometric exercises are started after 2 weeks.
Complications of graft dislodgment include difficulty swallowing and a sense of fullness in the throat.

Lumbar laminectomy for disk removal

DESCRIPTION ■ Removal of a disk from the intervertebral space.

INDICATIONS ■ Herniated nucleus pulposus (Fig. 7-3), sciatic pain more severe than chronic low back pain, positive lesègue sign, or neurologic deficit.

EQUIPMENT AND INSTRUMENTATION ■
Lumbar laminectomy instruments
Bipolar electrosurgical forceps
Positioning frame and/or pads, bolsters
Microscope for microdiscectomy

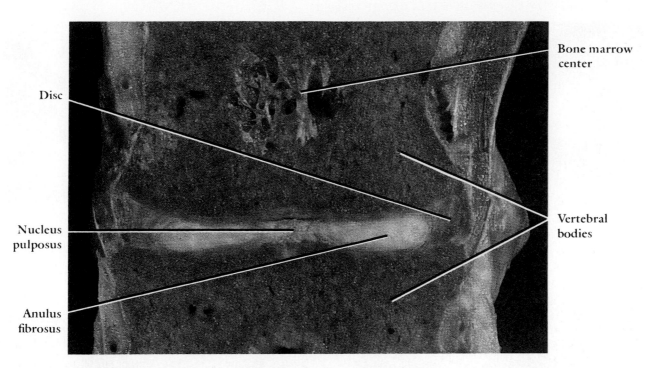

Disc

Nucleus
pulposus

Anulus
fibrosus

Bone marrow
center

Vertebral
bodies

Fig. 7-3 Lumbar vertebrae showing herniated nucleus pulposus. (From Vidic B, Suarez FR: *Photographic atlas of the human body*, St Louis, 1984, Mosby.)

PROCEDURE ■

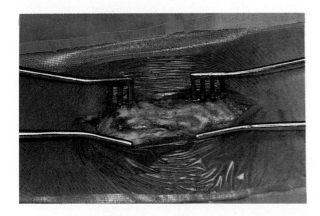

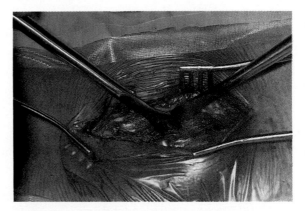

1 The patient is positioned prone on chest rolls or in the knee-chest position using a positioning frame, such as a Hastings, Hicks, or Andrews frame. The skin is prepared from the midthoracic region to the coccyx. A midline vertical incision is made at the operative site. The fascia is incised in the midline with a cautery or knife blade.

2 One side of the spinous processes, then the laminae, are exposed subperiosteally by sharp dissection using a Cobb elevator.

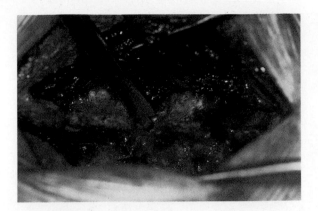

3 A partial hemilaminectomy of the laminal edges overlying the interspace of the herniated disk is performed using a rongeur or high-speed drill.

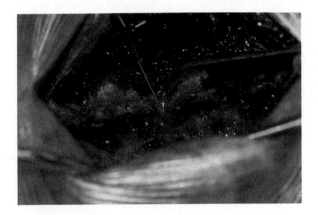

4 The ligamentum flava is incised using a No. 15 blade.

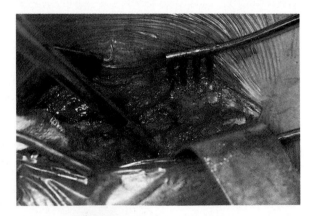

5 After the underlying dura is protected, additional ligament and/or the medial facet is removed, exposing the lateral recess to facilitate disk removal.

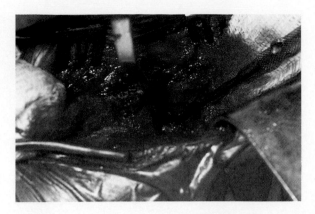

6 A dural elevator or nerve root retractor is used to retract the nerve root to expose the disk space; the extruded disk fragment is removed using a pituitary rongeur (not shown).

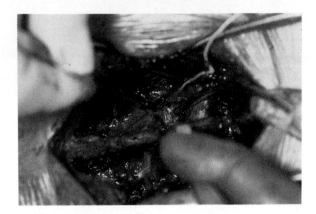

7 An opening is cut into the posterior aspect of the interspace with a No. 11 knife blade.

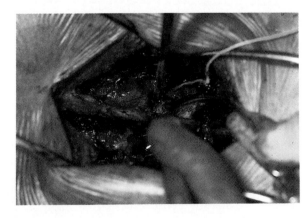

8 Disk material is removed from the interspace using a pituitary rongeur.

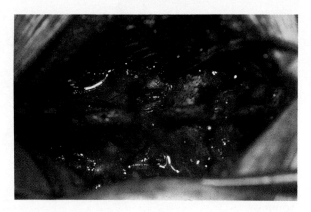

9 The foramen and extradural space are explored with a nerve hook or a ball-ended dissector.

10 The fascia, subcutaneous tissue, and skin are closed in layers.

■ NURSING CARE AND TEACHING CONSIDERATIONS ■

Encourage ambulation immediately.
Institute isometric abdominal and lower extremity exercises.
Provide patient instruction:
- Sitting and riding in a vehicle should be minimized.
- Lifting, bending, and stooping are prohibited for at least 2 weeks. Gradual introduction of lifting activities is begun after 6 weeks.
- If employed in a job that requires lifting, bending, and stooping, the patient is advised to remain off work for 6 weeks.

ARTHROPLASTY

Arthroplasty has become a common procedure for joint replacement necessitated by degenerative disease, fracture, or other cause of change in the joint. Prostheses resemble the anatomic structure being replaced.

Osteoarthritis is a degenerative condition associated with aging and causes tissue change in and around joints. It is the most common form of arthritis. The primary musculoskeletal tissues involved are the multiple layers of cartilage covering the ends of bones. As the cartilage deteriorates, other joint tissues are affected, leading to the symptoms of the degenerative disease.

Osteoarthritis appears as uneven, eroded surfaces resulting from deterioration of cartilage. This may be caused by stress on joints weakened by aging or may be secondary to trauma. Reattachments of detached cartilage into the joint may cause a chronic inflammation within the joint or the synovial lining. As articular cartilage continues to degenerate, the underlying bone produces spurs of bone, called osteophytes. These may also affect joint mobility and cause pain or discomfort as they increase in size. The major weight-bearing joints, such as the hip or knee, are the most commonly affected. Joints of the fingers, shoulder, elbow, wrist, and ankle may all be affected. Structures that cannot be replaced when these degenerative changes occur are the vertebrae, facet joints, and sacroiliac joints.

Rheumatoid arthritis is a systemic disease affecting many organs and the synovial lining of the joints. Joint inflammation is marked by edema, tenderness, pain, and limited motion. The synovium thickens and proliferates as inflammatory changes occur. Inflammatory changes lead to deterioration of the cartilage, leaving exposed bone surfaces. The most frequently affected joints are those of the hands, wrists, feet, ankles, and knees.

The type of implant selected for a procedure depends on the patient's condition or injury, the availability of the implant, and the physician's familiarity with the procedure. Custom implants are used for some conditions to mimic biomechanical characteristics.

Fixation means used in the implantation of joint prostheses include bone cement, porous fixation, and press fit. Bone cement is widely used. Porous fixation allows for tissue attachment using metallic substances with porous metallic coatings. Press fit has some provision for macrointerlock with bone, some with roughened surfaces and others with smooth surfaces. Descriptions of implants and the corresponding procedures are available from product representatives.

Metacarpophalangeal joint implant arthroplasty

DESCRIPTION ■ Use of a finger joint implant in combination with resection arthroplasty of the metacarpophalangeal (MP), proximal interphalangeal (PIP), and distal interphalangeal (DIP) joints. The implant maintains alignment and spacing of the reconstructed joint. It becomes encapsulated, stabilizing the implant. The stability of the joint is accomplished by reconstructing the ligamentous and musculotendinous systems.

INDICATIONS ■ Rheumatoid or traumatic arthritis, fixed or stiff MP joints, joint destruction or subluxation, or contracted muscles and ligaments.

EQUIPMENT AND INSTRUMENTATION ■
Soft tissue instruments
Small-bone instruments
Instrumentation for implants
Implants
Tourniquet
Hand table
Power equipment

PROCEDURE ■

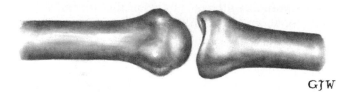

1 A transverse skin incision is made on the dorsum of the hand over the metacarpals. Using tenotomy scissors, dissection is carried out through the subcutaneous tissue, exposing the extensor tendons. Small retractors are used for exposure. The joint is exposed, and the head of the metacarpal is identified. An osteotome is used to transect the neck of the metacarpal. A pituitary rongeur may be used to remove synovia of the joint cavity and surrounding tissues. Soft tissue is released using the tenotomy scissors. A blunt hook may be used to pull up the tendons.

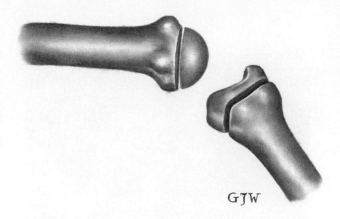

2 The base of the proximal phalanx is resected using a rongeur.

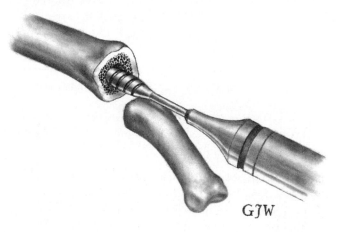

3 The intramedullary canal of the metacarpal is prepared using a rasp, a curette, and a power drill with a bur.

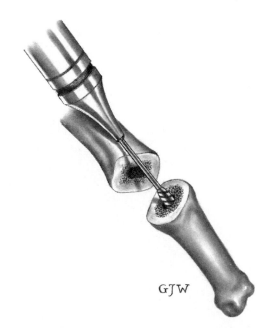

4 A hole is made at the base of the proximal phalanx, and the intramedullary canal is reamed using a bur, a reamer, and a curette.

5 Before the implant is inserted, holes may be placed for reattachment of the ligament. This improves the stability of the joint.

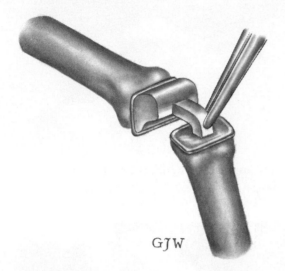

GJW

6 Sizers are used to determine the appropriate-size implant. The implant is placed. Implants are handled with blunt instruments to prevent damage.

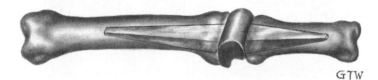

GJW

7 The skin incision is closed with a small subcuticular stitch (4-0 or 5-0 nylon). A dressing of sufficient size is applied to protect the hand. A narrow splint is placed on the palmar aspect of the hand and wrapped with a conforming bandage.

■ **NURSING CARE AND TEACHING CONSIDERATIONS** ■

Immediate and continuous elevation of the hand is required.
The dressing is replaced on the fifth postoperative day; the splint is maintained.
Exercises are started at 3 days postoperatively; full range of motion may not return.

Total elbow joint arthroplasty

DESCRIPTION ■ Replacement of the elbow joint with an implant.

INDICATIONS ■ Painful joint movement due to arthritis (rheumatoid or degenerative), loss of motion, trauma, instability, bone loss due to arthritis or trauma, or need for revision of a previously implanted prosthesis.

EQUIPMENT AND INSTRUMENTATION ■
Soft tissue instruments
Large-bone instruments
Instrumentation for implant
Implant
Tourniquet
Cement, mixer, and evacuator
Positioning equipment

PROCEDURE ■

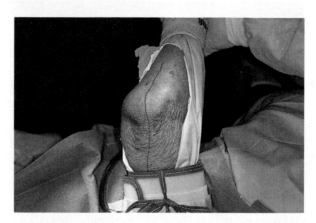

1 The patient may be positioned supine with a sandbag beneath the scapula and the arm across the chest. The lateral decubitus position may also be used. The elbow is draped free, and a sterile tourniquet is placed. The incision site is marked.

2 Following the initial skin incision, a cautery is used for dissection and to control bleeding.

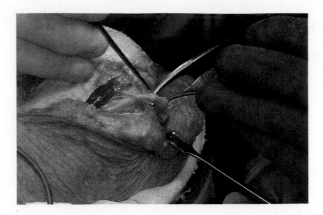

3 Senn retractors are used; dissection continues using Metzenbaum scissors to identify the triceps mechanism and ulnar nerve. The nerve is translocated anteriorly and protected throughout the remainder of the procedure.

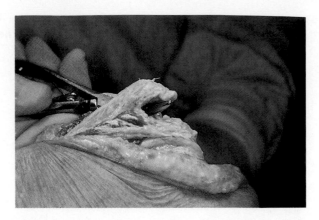

6 The ulnar periosteum is elevated along the forearm fascia.

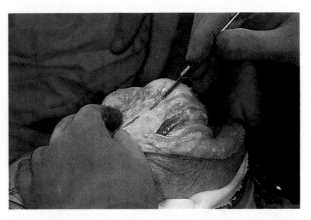

4 An incision is made over the medial aspect of the proximal ulna using a No. 10 blade.

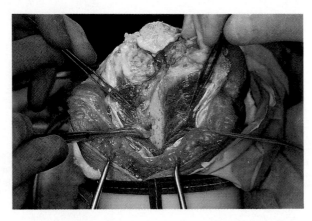

7 The extensor mechanism is subluxed laterally, allowing complete exposure of the distal humerus, proximal ulna, and radial head.

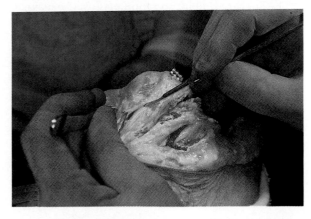

5 The triceps is removed from the proximal ulna by releasing Sharpey's fibers from their insertion using a blade, allowing release of the triceps.

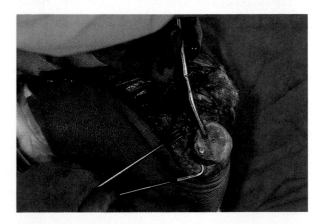

8 The tip of the olecranon is removed or notched to allow serial reamers to be introduced down the medullary canal.

9 The ulna is prepared by using a high-speed bur to remove subchondral bone. This allows introduction of serial reamers down the medullary canal.

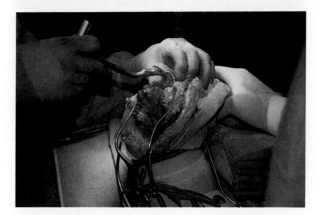

10 The appropriate-size rasp is used.

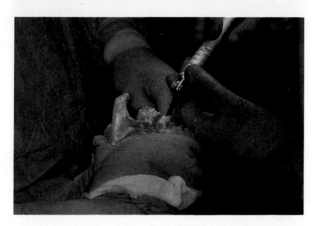

11 The midportion of the trochlea (distal humerus) is removed using an oscillating blade.

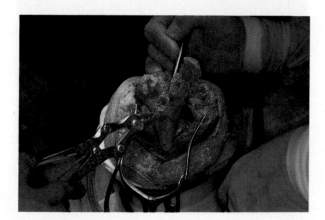

12 A Leksell rongeur is used to remove excess bony tissue caused by synovitis.

13 A bur is used to enter the roof of the olecranon fossa.

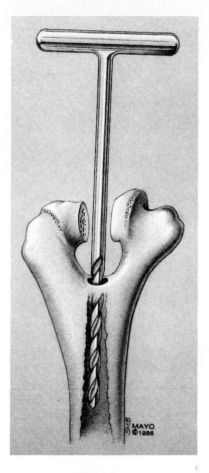

14 The medullary canal of the humerus is identified with a twist reamer.*

---

*Illustration reprinted by permission of Mayo Foundation.

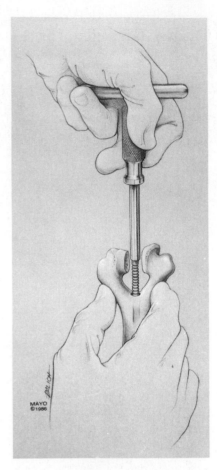

15 An alignment stem is placed down the canal of the humerus.*

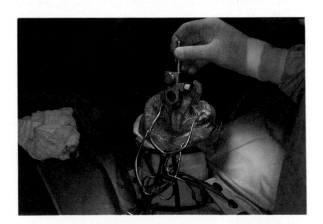

16 A humeral cutting guide is used to determine the appropriate depth of the cut.

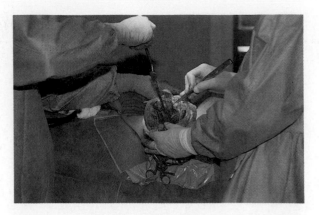

17 Rasps are inserted in a series of increasing size to prepare for the appropriate-size humeral component.

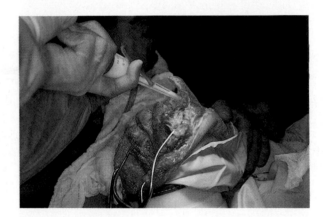

18 The medullary cavities of both bones are cleansed and dried. Cement is prepared and injected down the medullary canal of the ulna.

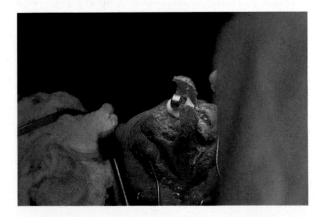

19 The ulnar component is cemented in place.

*Illustration reprinted by permission of Mayo Foundation.

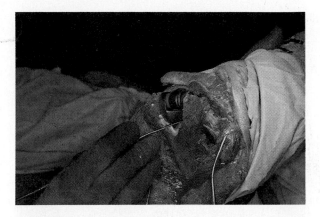

20 Following placement of the humeral component, excess cement is removed using a Freer elevator. The extremity is held in extension until the cement is hardened.

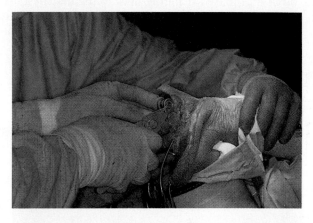

21 Split locking rings are placed to secure the component.

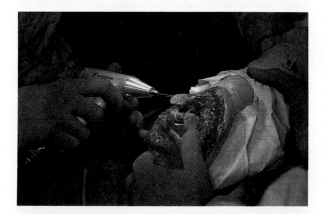

22 Holes are drilled in the proximal ulna for suturing the triceps mechanism in its anatomic position.

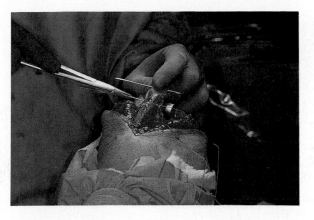

23 A Keith needle and Ethibond suture are used to secure the triceps.

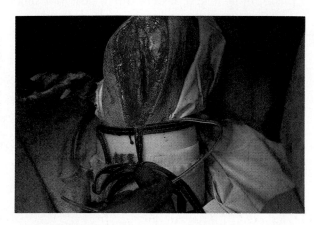

24 The tourniquet is deflated, and hemostasis is obtained. A Hemovac drain is placed.

25 The incision is closed in layers, and staples are placed in the skin.

26 A contact layer of dressing is applied, followed by an intermediate layer of dressing sponges. A compression dressing is applied with the elbow in full extension.

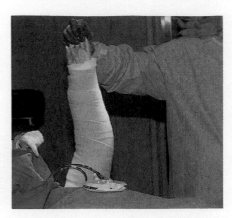

27 A ten-ply plaster splint is placed anteriorly to avoid pressure on the incision line. (The elbow can also be placed in 90-degree flexion with a posterior splint.) The dressing is secured with an elastic bandage.

> ■ **NURSING CARE AND TEACHING CONSIDERATIONS** ■
>
> Teaching includes short- and long-term postoperative restrictions. The patient is advised to lift no more than 1 pound over the next 3 months and to lift less than 5 pounds long term.
>
> The arm should remain elevated as much as possible for 4 or 5 days.
>
> Drains are removed at approximately 24 to 36 hours postoperatively.
>
> The dressing is removed on the third to fifth day postoperatively. Elbow flexion and extension, as tolerated, are allowed at this time.
>
> Physical therapy is not required. Occupational therapy for activities of daily living is indicated.

Shoulder joint arthroplasty

DESCRIPTION ■ Prosthetic replacement of the glenohumeral joint (the synovial ball-and-socket joint of the shoulder).

INDICATIONS ■ Osteoarthritis, rheumatoid arthritis, posttraumatic conditions (such as four-part displaced fractures or fracture dislocations), avascular necrosis, or neoplastic disease.

EQUIPMENT AND INSTRUMENTATION ■
Soft tissue instruments
Large-bone instruments
Shoulder instruments
Instrumentation for implant
Implant
Cement, mixer, and evacuator
Positioning equipment to elevate shoulder

PROCEDURE ■

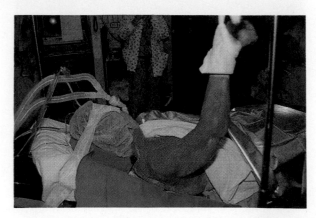

1 The patient is placed in a semisitting position with the affected shoulder near the edge of the bed. The area is prepared from the neck to the midchest, anteriorly and posteriorly, including the extremity, to the wrist. During the preparation the arm is suspended.

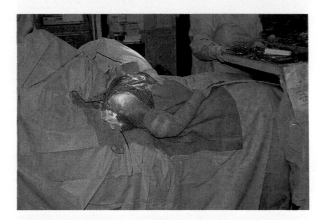

2 The arm is draped free to allow movement of the joint during the procedure.

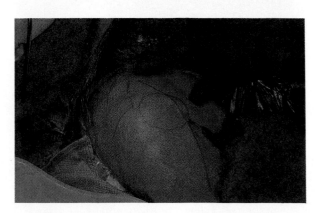

3 Using a No. 10 blade, an incision is made along the deltopectoral groove from the midacromion.

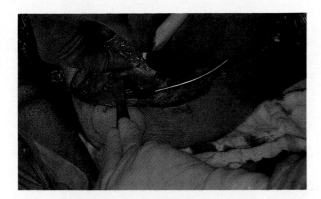

4 Dissection is carried out and hemostasis obtained using a cautery. Following identification of the cephalic vein, the deltopectoral interval is retracted using a Covell retractor. The superior margin of the pectoralis major is separated using a cautery.

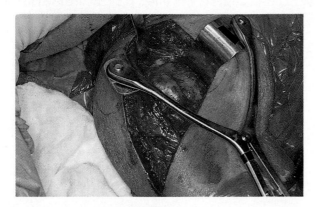

5 A Garra retractor is placed to retract the biceps tendon. A biceps tendon that is not intact is detached and will be attached in the bicipital groove before closure.

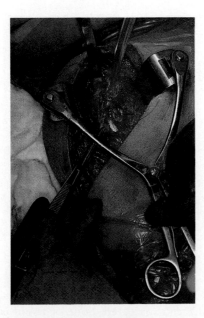

6 The subscapularis is divided.

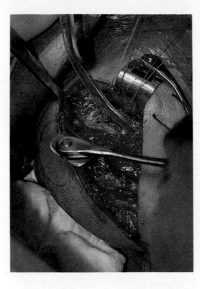

7 The subscapularis is retracted medially with Ethibond stay sutures to expose the interior of the joint.

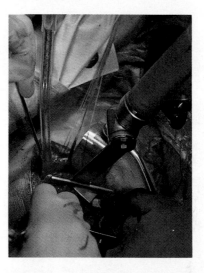

8 An osteotomy is performed using an oscillating saw blade along the guide at the anatomic neck.

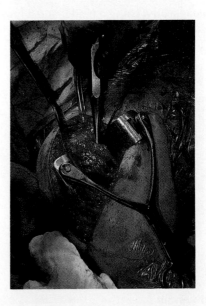

9 Following location of the canal of the humerus using a bur, the canal is cleaned with a curette.

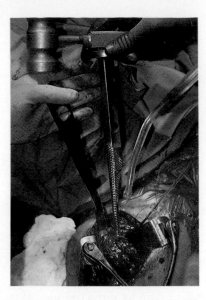

10 The shaft of the humerus is prepared using a hand-held reamer and mallet. Rasps are used in sequential order.

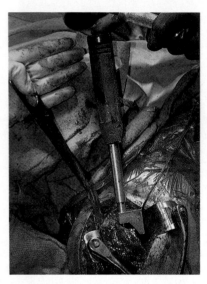

11 The trial is seated using a mallet and a humeral stem inserter.

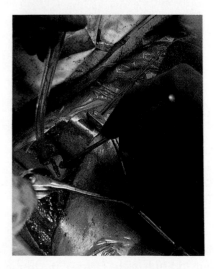

12 The glenoid fin cutting guide is inserted.

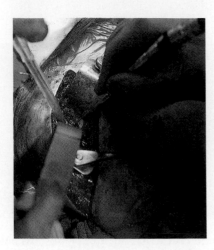

13 A small vertical groove is created through the center of the glenoid.

14 The saw, osteotomes, and a rongeur are used to trim osteophytes or protruding bone.

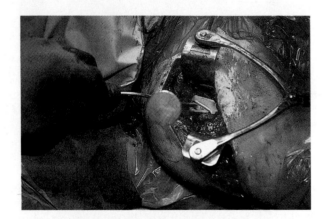

15 The glenoid fin rasp is used to enlarge the slot.

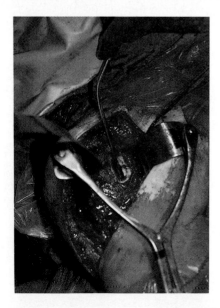

16 The surface is irrigated, bone or blood is removed, and the glenoid slot is dried.

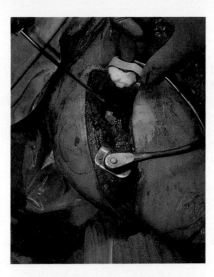

17 Bone cement is placed for glenoid insertion.

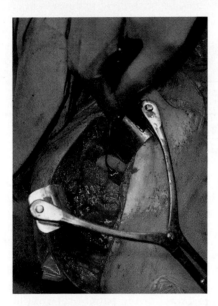

18 The glenoid is inserted. Cement is removed using a curette and ball-ended elevator.

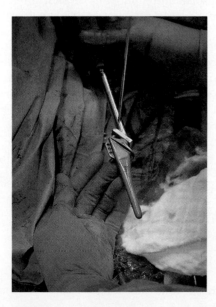

19 The humeral stem is placed using the inserter.

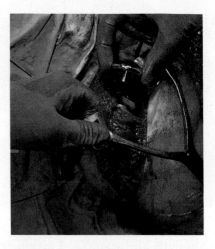

20 The humeral head is placed.

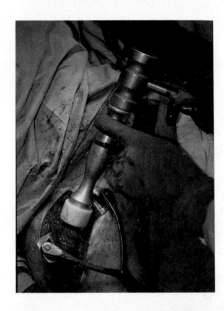

21 The implant is seated using the mallet.

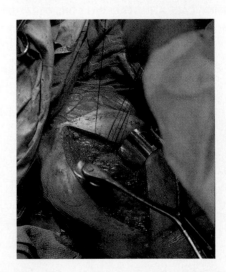

22 The subscapularis is closed with a nonabsorbable suture. Subscapularis tendon lengthening may be performed.

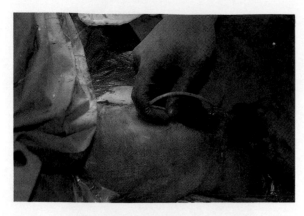

23 A Hemovac drain is placed between the deltoid and the rotator cuff. The wound is closed in layers.

24 A dressing of Steri-Strips, an intermediate layer, and tape is applied.

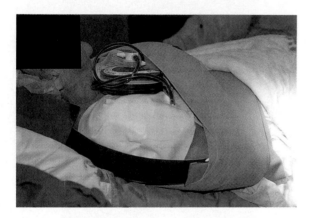

25 A postoperative sling is placed for immobilization. The specific condition of the patient may require modification of the postoperative dressing.

■ NURSING CARE AND TEACHING CONSIDERATIONS ■

The patient is assessed for willingness to participate in a vigorous program for up to 1 year.

Immobilization in the sling is continued for 1 to 2 days; then the sling is removed during the day as tolerated and used at night.

Passive exercises of forward flexion and external rotation are performed five times a day for 15 to 20 minutes.

Pendulum exercises are started at 1 to 10 days postoperatively.

Beginning with the second week, strengthening exercises are performed for 6 weeks.

Limits of external rotation are determined by preoperative ability.

Prosthetic replacement for a fracture

PROCEDURE ■ Following Step 6:

1 Bone-holding forceps are used to bring the greater tuberosity superiorly and anteriorly.

2 Holes are drilled in the humeral shaft and tuberosities. A No. 20 wire (or nonabsorbable suture) is passed for attachment of the tuberosities.

3 The shaft is prepared, and the implant is cemented.

4 The tuberosities are reattached.

5 Severe comminution or bone loss may require a bone graft.

■ NURSING CARE AND TEACHING CONSIDERATIONS ■

Passive movements should be started immediately, followed by assisted active mobilization.

Passive exercises are performed five times a day for 15 to 20 minutes.

Beginning the second week, strengthening exercises are performed for 6 weeks.

Hip arthroplasty (total hip replacement)

DESCRIPTION ■ Replacement of the acetabular cup and/or femoral head of the hip. Although the procedure described here involves a cemented implant, implants within the realm of total hip arthroplasty may also be noncemented and/or custom designed to meet individual patient and physician needs. Technical methods of replacement vary according to the implant used; product representatives can provide literature to inform operating room personnel of the patient care implications.

INDICATIONS ■ Degenerative or rheumatoid arthritis causing hip pain and immobility or pain at rest; congenital dysplasia of the hip; severe traumatic arthritis; or trauma.

Cemented implant: For older adults with osteoporosis and poor-quality bones (bones lack compressive strength to support weight-bearing forces; thin cortices may also lack the strength to resist the impaction forces of initial implant insertion).

Noncemented implant: For young, active individuals with strong, healthy bones. Requires bone stock adequate for fixation and the potential for new bone growth.

EQUIPMENT AND INSTRUMENTATION ■

Soft tissue instruments
Large-bone instruments
Instrumentation for implant
Implant
Cement, mixer, and evacuator
Bone plug
Power equipment
Positioning supplies

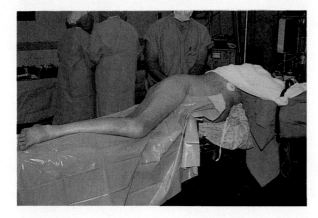

1   The patient is placed in a lateral position using a three-point positioner. A Vacpac can also be used to attain the lateral position (or another position may be selected). The arms are positioned on an armboard in anatomic alignment. The lower leg is bent slightly.

2   The area is prepared from the waist to the foot, including the groin and buttock. The leg is prepared circumferentially.

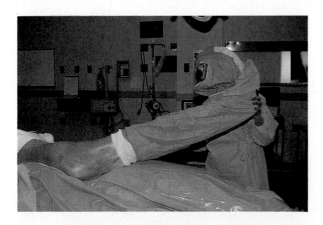

3   A sterile impervious ∪ drape is placed to occlude the perineum. Tails are applied to the back and stomach. A second ∪ drape is applied cephalad to the iliac crest. A stockinette is rolled over the foot to drape the lower extremity.

4   An elastic bandage is used to anchor the stockinette during the procedure.

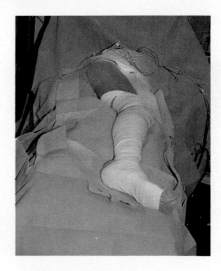

5   The extremity is draped free.

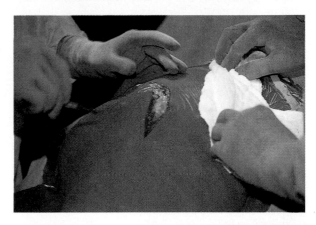

6   A lateral skin incision is made in line with the axis of the femur. Subcutaneous tissue is dissected from the fascial plane of the gluteus maximus and the tensor fascia lata. The incision should be large enough to expose the anatomic structures.

7   Femoral neck exposure is accomplished using sharp dissection with a No. 10 blade to identify and release the external rotators. A self-retaining Weitlaner retractor is placed.

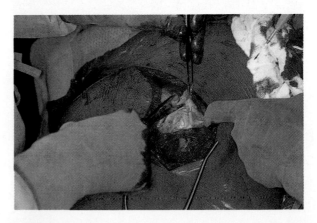

8   The bursa is dissected free using heavy scissors and forceps with teeth.

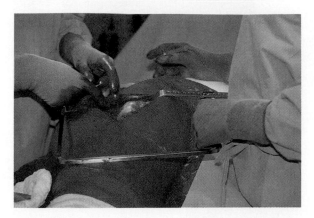

9 A self-retaining Charnley retractor is placed to provide exposure of the gluteus medius muscle attachment.

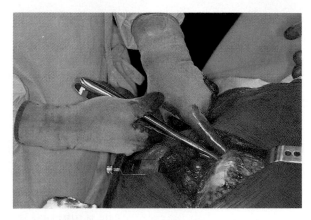

10 An Adson rongeur is used to remove fat and piriformis tendon.

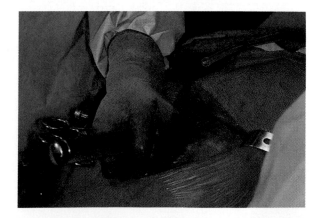

11 The head of the femur is levered and dislocated using a Cobb elevator.

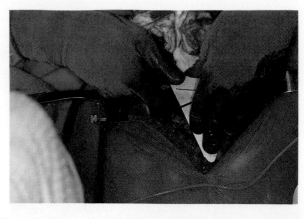

12 The femoral osteotomy guide is used to determine the location for transection of the femoral head and neck. A cautery is used to mark the level of the cut.

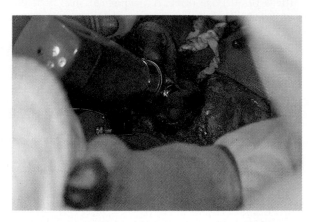

13 The osteotomy of the femoral neck is completed by cutting at the level of the collar using an oscillating saw blade.

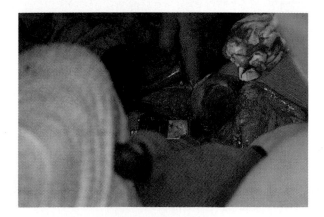

14 The femoral head is removed.

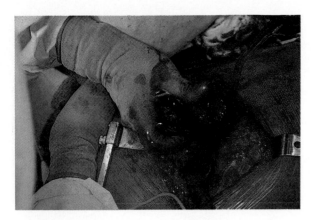

15 Soft tissue is removed from the acetabulum with a rongeur.

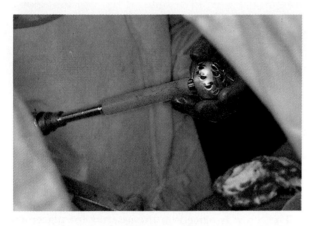

16 The reamer is assembled on the power equipment.

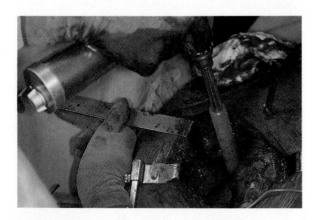

17 After the femoral head is removed, the acetabulum is exposed using an acetabular retractor and reamed.

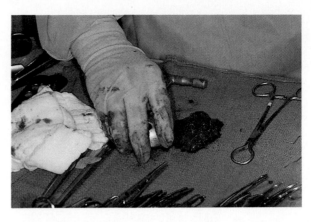

18 Retained acetabular bone from the reamers may be saved for bone grafting if needed.

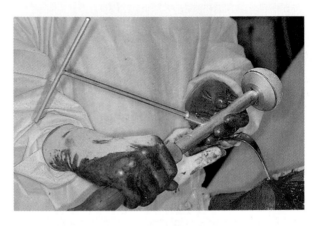

19 The correct-size implant is selected; it is positioned on the inserting device.

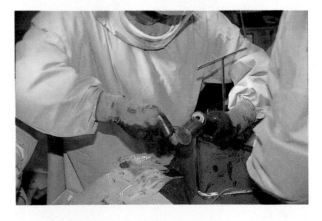

20 A mallet is used to seat the implant.

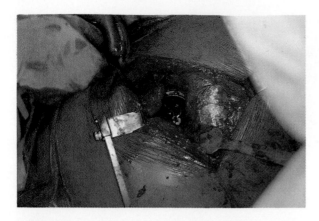

21   The prosthetic acetabulum liner is inserted.

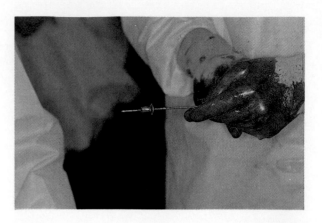

24   Screw length is determined using a depth gauge.

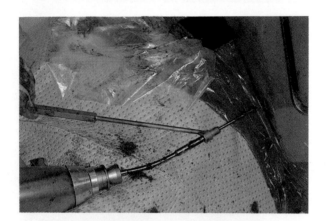

22   The screw guide is placed on the holder.

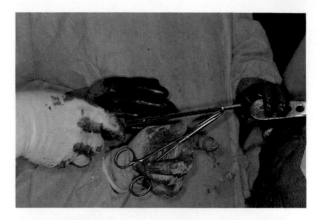

25   The screw is placed on the inserter for placement.

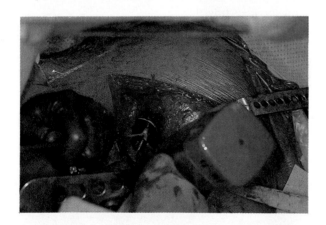

23   The acetabulum is drilled for screw placement.

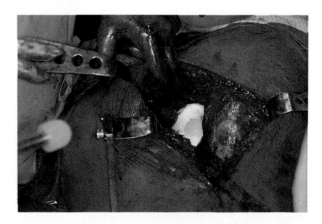

26   The acetabular liner is inserted.

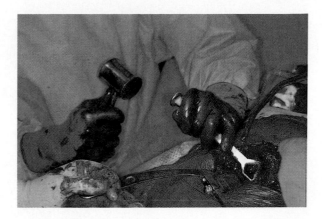

27 A box chisel is used to remove the remnant of the femoral neck.

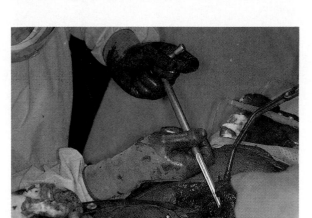

28 A hand-held tapered reamer starter is used to begin reaming.

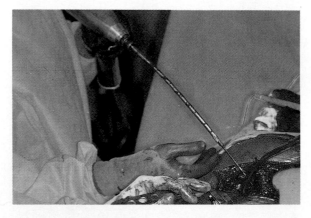

29 A flexible reamer is used for reaming. Straight intramedullary reamers are used to ream the canal.

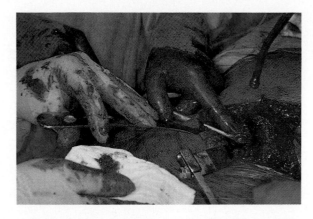

30 A large curette is used to remove bony tissue.

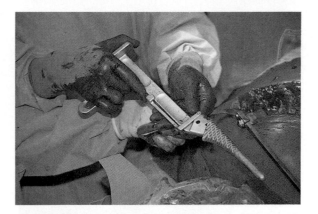

31 The implant is placed on the inserter.

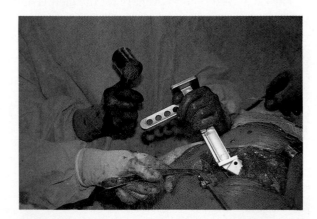

32 A broach and mallet are used to prepare the femoral canal.

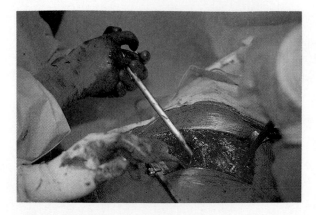

33 The trial is removed, and a cement plug is placed in the canal.

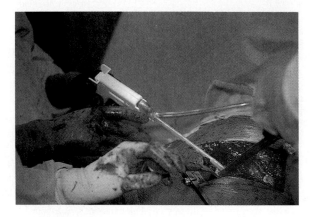

34 The canal is lavaged to prepare for the methyl methacrylate.

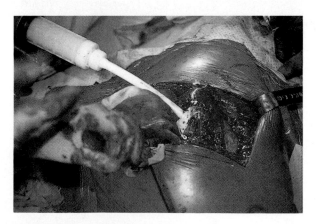

35 The cement (methyl methacrylate) is prepared and injected into the canal using a cement gun.

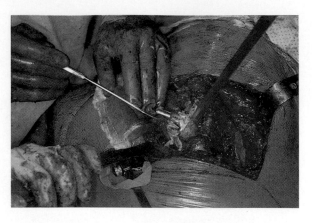

36 The femoral component of the implant is seated, and cement is removed from the edges of the implant.

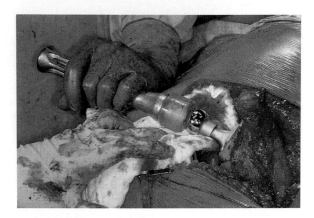

37 The head of the femoral component is placed using an impactor.

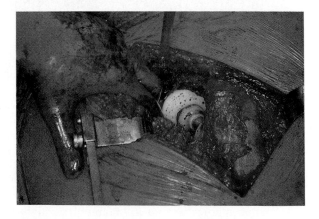

38 The hip is reduced after the cement has hardened.

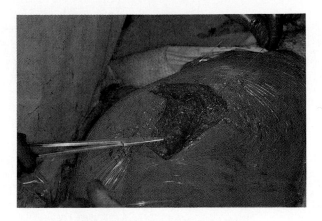

39 A drain is placed.

40 The incision site is closed with layers of absorbable suture.

41 Compression dressing is applied using a contact layer, intermediate layer, and tape. A hot ice pad is placed over the dressing, and an elastic bandage is used to secure the pad in place.

■ NURSING CARE AND TEACHING CONSIDERATIONS ■

Anticoagulant therapy may be used to prevent post-operative complications.
Passive motion exercises are started immediately.
Adduction of the hip may be required for up to 4 weeks postoperatively.
Non-weight-bearing, ambulation progressing to toe touch, may be maintained, depending on the reason for the implant, the patient's condition, and/or the type of implant.

Knee arthroplasty (total knee replacement)

DESCRIPTION ■ Cemented or noncemented prosthetic replacement of the femoral, tibial, and possibly the patellar components of the knee.

INDICATIONS ■ Pain and instability due to degenerative, rheumatoid, or traumatic arthritis; or medial or lateral compartment destruction due to extreme varus or valgus deformity.

EQUIPMENT AND INSTRUMENTATION ■
Soft tissue instruments
Large-bone instruments
Instrumentation for implant
Implant
Tourniquet
Power equipment
Cement, mixer, and evacuator
Positioning equipment

PROCEDURE ■

1 The patient is positioned supine with a tourniquet on the upper thigh. A leg holder is placed on the bed. The extremity is prepared circumferentially from the incision site. The leg is draped free, and a stockinette is placed over the foot. The leg holder is positioned, an elastic bandage is used to wrap the extremity, and an impervious drape is placed over the exposed skin.

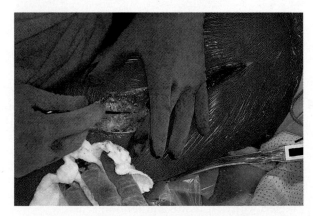

2 An anterior longitudinal incision is made over the knee using a No. 10 blade.

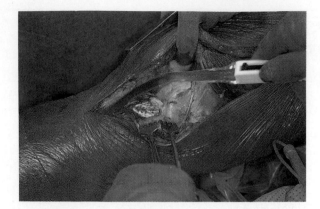

3 Subcutaneous tissue is dissected using an electrosurgical pencil (not shown) for hemostasis and cutting. Rake retractors are placed for exposure. The capsule is entered anteromedially, approximately 1 cm from the medial border of the patella, using a No. 10 blade. The patellar ligament is partially elevated medially. With exposure established, osteophytes are removed with a rongeur (not shown), and the patella is everted and dislocated laterally. Medial and lateral tibial plateaus are exposed.

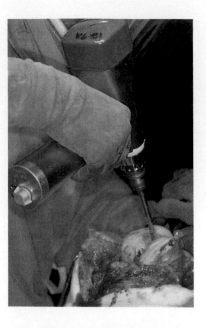

5 A hole is drilled in the center of the distal femur using the power equipment. Hohmann retractors are used for exposure.

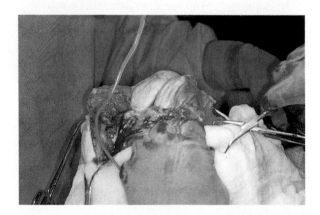

4 A portion of the infrapatellar fat pad is excised, and the tibia is subluxed; the plateau surfaces can now be visualized. Soft tissues such as the patellar fat pad, the anterior cruciate ligament, capsular bands or adhesions, and the attainable portions of the meniscus are resected using a No. 10 blade (or scissors). Fixed varus, fixed valgus, and fixed flexion are corrected with soft tissue and tendon releases.

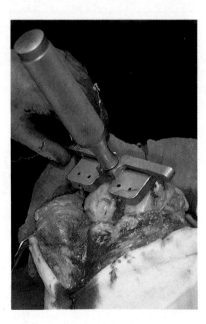

6 The femoral intramedullary alignment guide is positioned parallel with the femoral condyles.

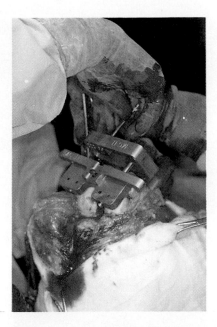

7 The anterior femoral cutting guide is placed, and pins are used to secure the guide.

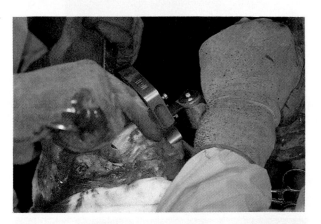

8 The femoral (distal and anterior) condyles are cut using an oscillating saw blade.

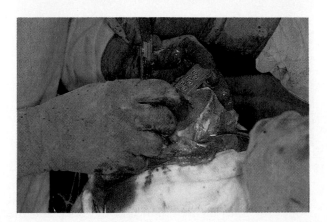

9 The anteroposterior measuring guide is placed for determining the size of the femoral component.

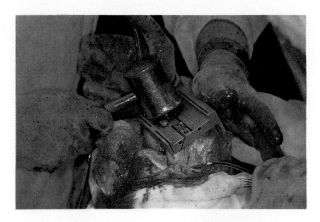

10 The distal femoral cutting guide is secured with two or three pins. A drill is used to make holes for the pins and the mallet, to complete pin placement.

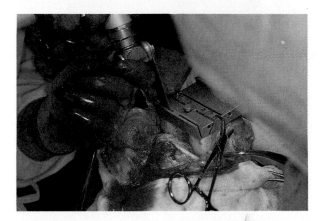

11 The distal femur is cut with the oscillating saw blade.

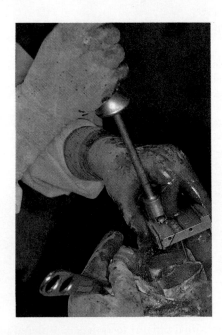

12 The pins are removed.

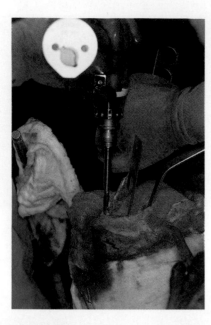

13 A drill hole is made in the proximal tibia.

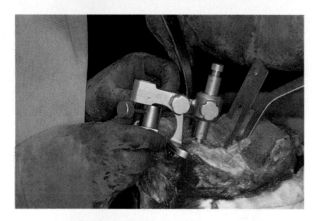

14 The components of the intramedullary tibial resector are assembled.

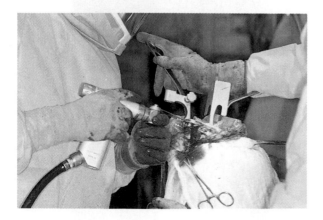

15 The proximal tibial resection is completed using the oscillating saw blade.

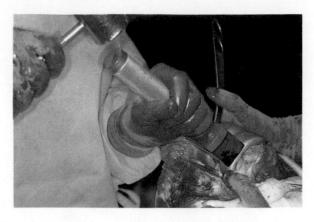

16 The femoral trial component is positioned.

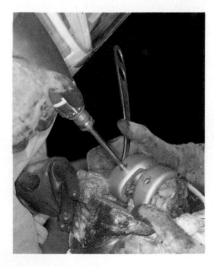

17 Drill holes are made.

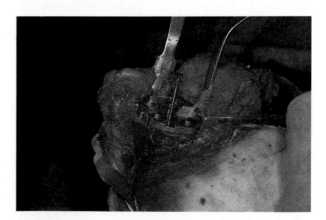

18 The tibial trial component is positioned. The knee is articulated and taken through its range of motion. If cement is to be used, it is prepared and placed onto the ends of the femur and the tibia, and the implants are inserted.

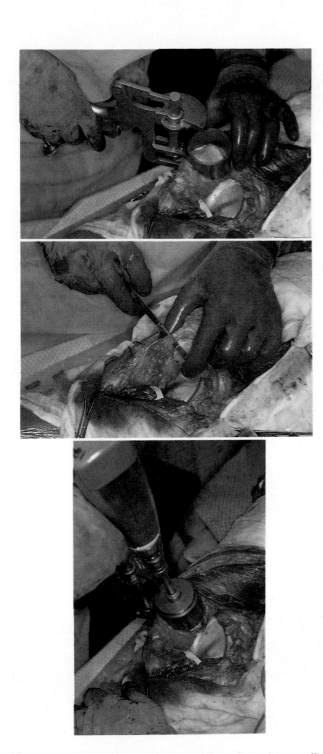

19 The patellar saw guide is positioned on the patella.

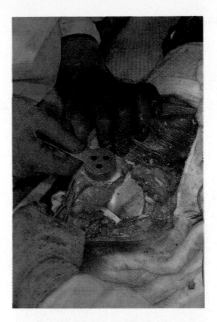

20 The patellar drill guide is positioned.

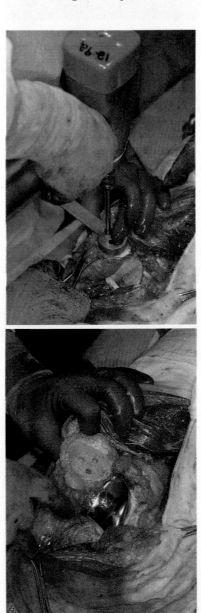

21 Holes are drilled in the patella.

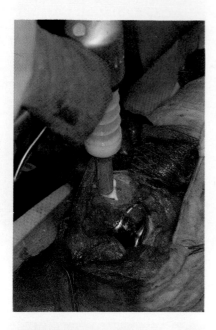

22   Cement is injected into the patellar holes.

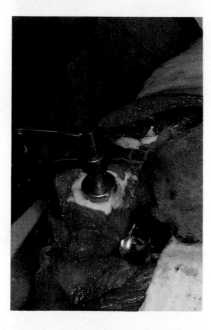

23   A polyethylene patellar button is cemented to the prepared patella. A patellar clamp is used to secure the patellar button until the cement hardens. Excess cement is removed.

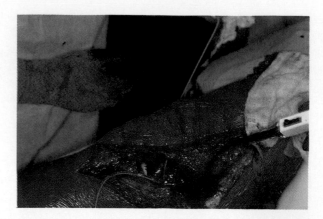

24   A closed wound suction drain is inserted, and the incision is closed.

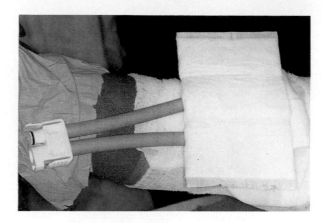

25   The contact and intermediate layers of dressing are applied, followed by a hot ice pack. A knee immobilizer is applied before the patient is extubated.

■ NURSING CARE AND TEACHING CONSIDERATIONS ■

Continuous passive motion is started immediately.
Restricted ambulation is started immediately; immediate weight-bearing ambulation is started if the components are cemented.
Crutch walking is started as soon as it is determined that weight bearing can be tolerated.
Strengthening exercises are started within 2 weeks.

PROCEDURES TO CORRECT DISORDERS OF THE FOOT

There are approximately 130 procedures for hallux valgus complexes, commonly called bunions. Hallux valgus is a complex deformity, appearing as a lateral deviation of the great toe with symptoms usually accompanying the lesser toes. In many cases it is considered a hereditary trait. Procedures for correction of this deformity include:

- Revision of soft structures
- Resection of bone or hemiarthroplasty
- Correction of varus deformity of the first metatarsal by osteotomy
- Correction of varus deformity of the first metatarsal by revision of the soft structures
- Correction of valgus deformity of the great toe by osteotomy of its proximal phalanx
- Arthrodesis of the first metatarsophalangeal joint

Chevron distal metatarsal osteotomy

DESCRIPTION ■ Correction of a valgus deformity of the first metatarsal by osteotomy.

INDICATIONS ■ Commonly performed in middle-aged patients with a hallux valgus angle of less than 40 degrees and an intermetatarsal angle (the angle between the first and second metatarsals) of less than 15 to 20 degrees.

EQUIPMENT AND INSTRUMENTATION ■
Small-bone instruments
Soft tissue instruments
Tourniquet
Small power saw, thin saw blade
Kirschner pin

PROCEDURE ■

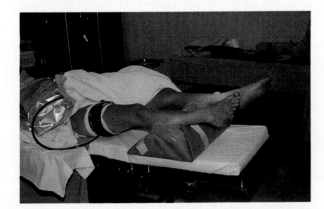

1 The patient is positioned supine with the extremities protected, and a tourniquet is placed on the upper thigh.

2 The surgical area is prepared from the foot to the ankle circumferentially, and the extremity is draped to expose the foot.

3 Using a No. 15 blade, a medial longitudinal skin incision is made over the medial metatarsophalangeal joint to the joint capsule.

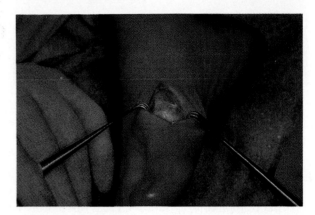

4 After the skin edges are retracted with double hooks or Senn rakes, soft tissue is stripped from the medial eminence using a No. 15 blade on a knife handle.

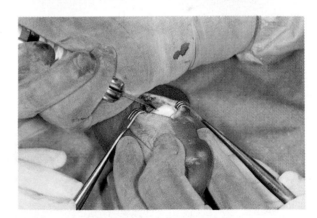

5 Using a small power saw with a thin blade (an osteotome can also be used), the medial eminence is excised.

6 The medial eminence is removed.

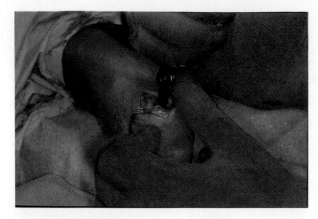

7 In the distal portion of the metatarsal head a Chevron osteotomy is made using a small power saw with a thin blade.

8 Using manual pressure (or towel clips) on the first metatarsal shaft and the first metatarsal head, the distal fragment is displaced laterally, effectively narrowing the forefoot.

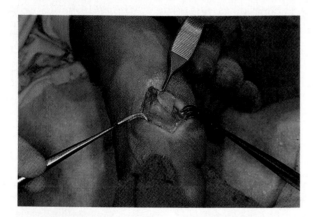

9 The excess portion of the metaphysis is removed using the saw.

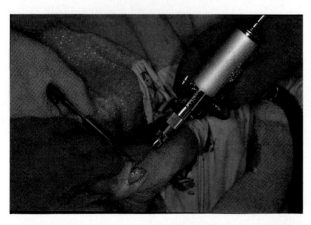

10 If necessary, a .062 smooth pin may be inserted to stabilize the osteotomy site.

11 While the great toe is held in the correct position, the medial capsule is closed snugly with a large-gauge absorbable suture.

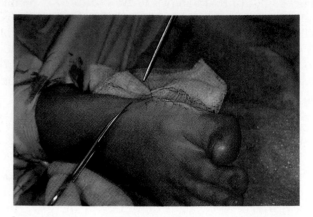

12 Skin closure is completed using a small-gauge (4-0 or 5-0) nonabsorbable suture.

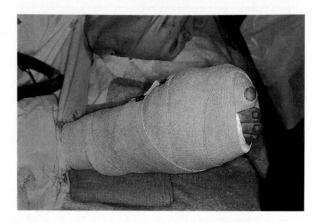

13 A soft compression dressing is applied.

■ **NURSING CARE AND TEACHING CONSIDERATIONS** ■

The foot should be elevated as much as possible.

With the patient wearing a postoperative shoe, ambulation is maintained at a minimal level for 2 weeks.

A round-toe athletic shoe or sandal is worn for 2 to 6 weeks.

A bunion splint is worn at night from the second to the sixth postoperative week.

Activities may be resumed in 6 weeks.

One-inch heels may be worn at 8 to 10 weeks postoperatively.

Physical therapy may be required for heel-toe gait and first metatarsal phalangeal movement.

Keller resection arthroplasty

DESCRIPTION ■ Medial eminence resection (bunionectomy) and resection of the base of the proximal phalanx for treatment of hallux valgus.

INDICATIONS ■ Impaired function due to symptoms; or cosmetic reasons.

EQUIPMENT AND INSTRUMENTATION ■
Small-bone instruments
Soft tissue instruments
Tourniquet
Small power saw, thin saw blade
Osteotomes

PROCEDURE ■

1 The patient is positioned supine, a tourniquet is placed on the upper thigh, the incision site is marked, and the skin preparation is completed. The extremity is draped free.

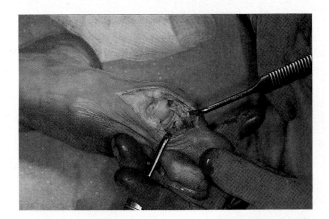

2 Following a medial capsular incision, the first metatarsophalangeal joint is exposed by dissecting the joint capsule and periosteum away from the medial aspect of the proximal phalanx. Swanson retractors are used to enhance exposure.

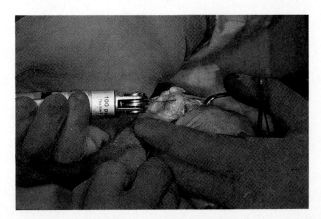

3 The medial eminence flare is removed using a small power saw blade (or a ½-inch osteotome).

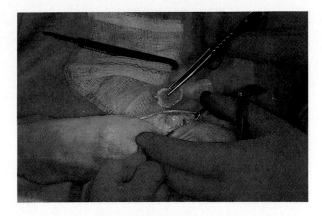

4 The medial eminence is removed.

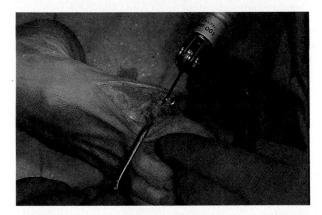

5 The proximal one-fourth to one-third aspect of the proximal phalanx is resected using a small power saw with a narrow blade (or ½-inch osteotome). Sharp margins of the osteotomy and osteophytes around the metatarsal head can be removed with a rongeur if necessary. (Not shown: holes can be made using a ⅛-inch drill bit on the medial and plantar aspects of the diaphysis of the proximal phalanx to reattach the medial capsule and plantar place to the proximal phalanx.)

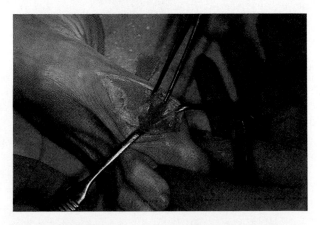

6 The proximal phalanx fragment is removed.

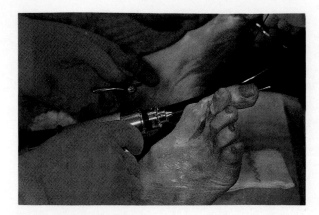

7 The toe is stabilized using a .062 pin inserted in a retrograde to antegrade direction across the first metatarsophalangeal joint into the first metatarsal head. The pin exits distally and is left percutaneous at the tip of the great toe.

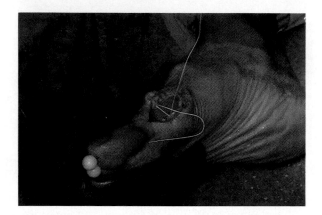

8 A snug capsular closure is completed using an appropriate-gauge absorbable suture, and the skin edges are reapproximated.

9 Closure is completed using a nonabsorbable suture. The pin is cut, and Jergens pin balls are applied.

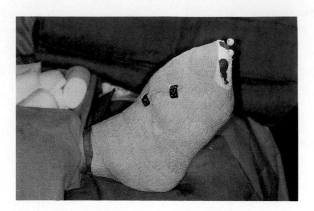

10 A soft compression dressing is applied.

■ NURSING CARE AND TEACHING CONSIDERATIONS ■

Non-weight-bearing ambulation should be maintained for 3 to 5 days.

The foot should be elevated as much as possible.

Dressing changes are done at 3 to 5 days postoperatively; suture removal is done at 10 to 14 days.

Ambulation should be minimal, with a postoperative shoe worn for the first 4 weeks.

Pins are removed after approximately 4 weeks.

Physical therapy may be required for heel-toe gait and flexion of joints.

High-impact exercise can be resumed after 6 to 8 weeks.

Hammertoe correction

DESCRIPTION ■ Excision of the distal end of the proximal phalanx.

INDICATIONS ■ Pain due to abnormal flexion of the proximal interphalangeal joint of one of the lesser four toes, described as hammertoe.

EQUIPMENT AND INSTRUMENTATION ■
Small-bone instruments
Soft tissue instruments
Small power saw
Kirschner pin

PROCEDURE ■

1 A tourniquet is placed on the upper thigh. The foot and leg are prepared to midcalf, and the extremity is draped free.

2 A longitudinal dorsal incision is made over the proximal interphalangeal joint using a No. 15 blade, splitting the extensor tendon.

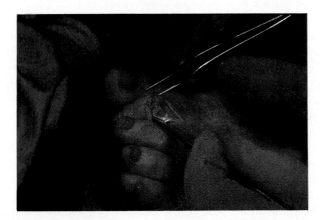

3 Skin edges are retracted (skin hooks can be used), and the collateral ligaments are released, exposing the distal end of the proximal phalanx.

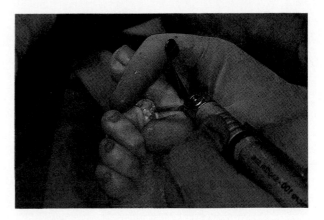

4 Excision of the distal end of the proximal phalanx is completed using a small power saw (or rongeur); a towel clip may be used to stabilize the distal end of the proximal phalanx during resection.

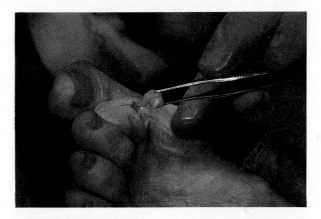

5 The proximal phalanx fragment is resected.

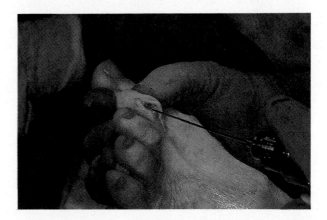

6 The toe is then stabilized, if necessary, using a smooth .045 Kirschner pin. A small-gauge absorbable suture may be used to reapproximate the extensor mechanism.

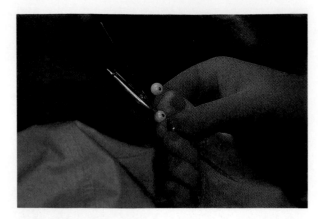

7 A pin cutter is used to remove excess pin, and a Jergens pin ball is applied. The skin edges are closed using a small-gauge nonabsorbable suture.

8 A soft dressing is applied.

■ NURSING CARE AND TEACHING CONSIDERATIONS ■

The foot should be elevated as much as possible.
The patient should remain on bed rest for 1 to 3 days.
Dressings are changed at 3 to 5 days postoperatively.
A dry foot is maintained until the pins are (removed at 2 to 6 weeks); showering should be avoided.
Ambulation should be minimal for 6 weeks postoperatively.
A postoperative walking shoe should be worn until the pins are removed at (2 to 6 weeks).
Nonimpact exercise is allowed after 2 weeks, higher-impact exercise is allowed at 6 weeks.

BONE GRAFT AND STIMULATION

Bone graft material can add three essential properties to the host tissue bed to enhance bone healing: osteogenic potential, osteoconductive potential, and osteoinductive properties (Table 7-1). Preparation of the bony surface is a matter of preference and is dictated by the method of internal fixation.

Osteogenic potential is the ability of the graft material to make bone. Autogenous bone and bone marrow are osteogenic graft materials. Osteoconductivity is the property of the graft material that facilitates the bone-healing response so that the response is distributed uniformly over the tissue volume in which the graft is placed. Osteoconductive materials include purified fibrillar collagen, bone and bone matrix, and some ceramics, such as hydroxyapatite and tricalcium phospate. Osteoinduction is the process by which some stimulus "induces" bone growth, as exhibited by at least one protein in bone matrix, bone morphogenetic protein (BMP). Three types of bone grafts are available: autogenous, from the patient's own body; allografts (homografts), from individuals other than the patient; and xenografts (heterografts), from other species.

Autogenous cancellous bone is currently the most successful bone graft material. It combines osteogenic, osteoconductive, and osteoinductive properties. It differs from cortical bone in the rate, mechanism, and completeness of repair. Disadvantages of autogenous graft harvest include added operative time, blood loss, and operative trauma. The amount of autogenous bone is also sometimes limited.

Autogenous cortical bone grafts have traditionally been found to be less successful than cancellous grafts. The advantage of cortical bone over the other graft materials is its mechanical strength.

Allograft is tissue transplanted from one individual to another member of the same species. The demand for musculoskeletal tissues such as bone, cartilage, and ligaments has increased. Tissue banks have been established in the United States to provide graft materials that are obtained surgically under aseptic conditions. Successful bone banking requires meticulous

Table 7-1 ■ *Properties of bone graft materials*

	Osteoinductive	Osteoconductive	Osteogenic
Autogenous bone	X	X	X
Alloimplant bone	X	X	
Bone marrow			X
Bone matrix	X	X	
BMP	X		

quality control and standardized, reproducible methods of tissue processing. Freezing and freeze-drying (lyophilization) are the most commonly used methods of preparation. Freeze-drying may result in as much as 50% reduction in mechanical strength because of changes in biomechanical properties. Sterilization methods include irradiation and gas autoclaving with ethylene oxide.

Bone graft

DESCRIPTION ▪ Bone taken from a surgical site other than where the operative procedure is being completed.

INDICATIONS ▪ Nonunion, delayed union, congenital pseudoarthrosis, or bone defects.

EQUIPMENT AND INSTRUMENTATION ▪
Soft tissue instruments
Elevators: periosteal or Cobb
Gouges
Curettes
Osteotomes

Cancellous bone graft—iliac crest
PROCEDURE ▪

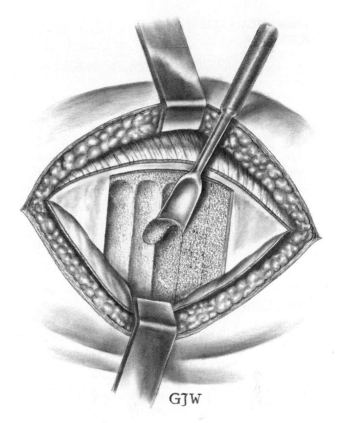

2 Cancellous bone is obtained using curettes and/or gouges.

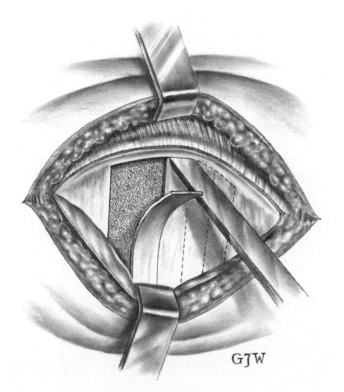

1 An incision is made along the border of the iliac crest. The incision is extended through the muscles to the iliac crest. The crest is stripped with Cobb elevator(s), or a cortical window is made using osteotomes and a mallet. Strips of the crest are removed using a ½-inch osteotome and the mallet.

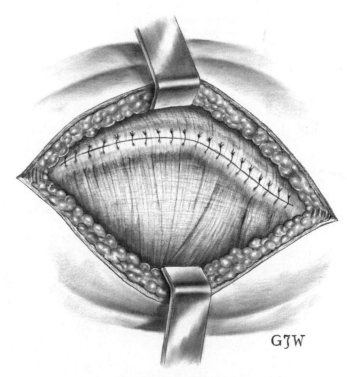

3 Bone wax may be applied to decrease bleeding. The incision is closed using an absorbable suture.

Cortical bone graft—tibia
PROCEDURE ■

1 A curved anteromedial incision is made along the tibia.
2 The periosteum is incised with an osteotome and reflected.
3 The graft site is outlined with drill holes using a drill bit.
4 The graft is removed with a ½-inch osteotome. An oscillating bone saw blade can also be used.

■ NURSING CARE AND TEACHING CONSIDERATIONS ■

Observe the incision dressing for bleeding.

Bone stimulation

DESCRIPTION ■ An alternative method of treatment alone or as an adjunct to surgery for promotion of bone union. Details of the electrophysiologic properties of bone have not been ascertained, but the response of bone to invasive and noninvasive electrical signals has led to the development of devices for this purpose. Bone growth can be enhanced by use of an electrode, an electric field, or an induced electric current to influence or induce osteogenesis.

INDICATIONS ■ Nonunion, delayed union, congenital pseudoarthrosis, or bone defects.

EQUIPMENT AND INSTRUMENTATION ■
Two types of implantable direct-current stimulators are available. The invasive system requires implantation with the patient anesthetized. Components include a small generator, lead wires, and a cathode.
Soft tissue instruments.

Insertion of a long-bone stimulator
PROCEDURE ■

1 The bone requiring an implant is exposed using soft tissue instruments.
2 The canal on either side of the nonunion is formed using a curette, drill, or rasp to ensure medullary canal continuity.

3 The cathode wire is placed in the defect.
4 A second incision is made 8 to 10 cm from the nonunion site. A tunnel is made in the subcutaneous tissue using digital dissection or a hemostat. Hemostasis is attained.
5 The generator is implanted beneath the deep fascia. The cathode lead is directed through the tunnel.
6 A bone graft may be necessary if a large bony defect is being treated.
7 The incision site is closed.

Benefits of the stimulator are recognized for up to 8 months; at that time the generator is the only portion removed.

Insertion of a fusion site stimulator
PROCEDURE ■ Before the fusion site is closed, four electrodes of the stimulator are implanted. The stimulation is effective for up to 16 weeks. Removal of the device is required.

Noninvasive stimulation
PROCEDURE ■ Noninvasive stimulators are applied to the skin in the area requiring therapy.

Inductive stimulation is a noninvasive form of therapy that creates a magnetic field around the nonunion or fusion site. The inductive stimulators currently being marketed function using battery power that requires recharging. Daily treatments of 3 to 10 hours a day are required for approximately 6 months. Treatment results are often related to patient compliance.

Capacitive coupled stimulation relies on the production of an electrical field by means of an external capacitor. One form is on the market, but it is not indicated for use in the spine.

■ NURSING CARE AND TEACHING CONSIDERATIONS ■

Patient response to therapy and compliance may be related to anxiety.
Patient teaching and reinforcement is critical to encouraging compliance.

BIBLIOGRAPHY

Association of Operating Room Nurses, Inc.: *AORN standards and recommended practices for perioperative nursing—1992,* Denver, 1992, AORN.

Bordelon RL: Evaluation and operative procedures for hallux valgus deformity, *Orthopedics* 10:38, Jan 1987.

Brazytis KE, Hergenroeder P: Arthroscopic ankle surgery: overcoming anatomic difficulties with improved techniques, *AORN J* 55:492, Feb 1992.

Bucholz, RW and others: *Orthopaedic decision making,* St Louis, 1984, Mosby.

Buckham K: Surgical bone banking: the living donor, *Orthop Nurs* 10:47, March/April 1991.

Burke KFD, McGrouther DA, Smith PJ: *Principles of hand surgery,* New York, 1990, Churchill Livingstone.

Cameron HU: *The technique of total hip arthroplasty,* St Louis, 1992, Mosby.

Canale ST, Beaty JH: *Operative pediatric orthopaedics,* St Louis, 1991, Mosby.

Carter R: *The shoulder,* New York, 1988, Churchill Livingstone.

Chapman MW: *Operative orthopedics,* vols 1 and 2, Philadelphia, 1988, JB Lippincott.

Colton CL, Hall AJ: *Atlas of orthopedic surgical approaches,* Oxford, 1991, Butterworth/Heinemann.

Crenshaw AH: *Campbell's operative orthopaedics,* vols 1 to 5, ed 8, St Louis, 1992, Mosby.

Doyle JR: Anatomy of the finger flexor tendon sheath and pulley system, *J Hand Surg* 13:473, 1988.

Evarts CM: *Surgery of the musculoskeletal system,* ed 2, New York, 1990, Churchill Livingstone.

Gartland J: *Fundamentals of orthopaedics,* ed 4, Philadelphia, 1987, WB Saunders.

Goldstein LA, Dickerson RC: *Atlas of orthopaedic surgery,* ed 2, St Louis, 1981, Mosby.

Gross T and others: The biology of bone grafting, *Orthopedics* 14:563, May 1991.

Hoshowsky V: Chronic lateral ligament instability of the ankle, *Orthop Nurs* 7:33, May/June 1988.

Laurin CA, Riley LH, Roy-Camille R: *Atlas of orthopaedic surgery,* vols 2 and 3, St Louis, 1989, 1992, Mosby.

May P: Dupuytren's contracture: surgical principles, nursing implications, *AORN J* 54:46, July 1991.

Meeker M, Rothrock J: *Alexander's care of the patient in surgery,* ed 9, St Louis, 1991, Mosby.

Mercier LR and others: *Practical orthopedics,* ed 3, St Louis, 1991, Mosby.

Morrey B: *Joint replacement arthroplasty,* New York, 1991, Churchill Livingstone.

Mourad LA: *Orthopaedic disorders,* St Louis, 1991, Mosby.

Nichols CS: Wrist arthroscopy: an ambulatory surgery procedure, *AORN J* 49:759, March 1989.

O'Connell WD: Video technology: basics for perioperative nurses, *AORN J* 56:442, Sept 1992.

Orr PM: An educational program for total hip and knee replacement patients as part of a total arthritis center program, *Orthop Nurs* 9:61, Sept/Oct 1990.

Paulos LE, Tibone JE: *Operative techniques in shoulder surgery,* Gaithersburg, Md, 1991, Aspen.

Paulos LE and others: Anterior cruciate ligament reconstruction with autografts, *Clin Sports Med* 10:469, July 1991.

Post M, Morrey BF, Hawkins RJ: *Surgery of the shoulder,* St Louis, 1990, Mosby.

Reckling FW, Reckling JB, Mohn MP: *Orthopaedic anatomy and surgical approaches,* St Louis, 1990, Mosby.

Rothrock JC: *Perioperative nursing care planning,* St Louis, 1990, Mosby.

Scott WN, Stillwell WT: *Arthroplasty: an atlas of surgical technique,* Rockville, Md, 1987, Aspen.

Sculco TP: *Orthopaedic care of the geriatric patient,* St Louis, 1985, Mosby.

Skinner HB: Alternatives in the selection of allograft bone, *Orthopedics* 13:843, Aug 1990.

Snyder S, Kelly K: Arthroscopic evaluation and treatment of rotator cuff pathology: a nursing perspective, *AORN J* 56:225, Aug 1992.

Spaulding Megesi RG and others: Total ankle arthroplasty: procedural review, *AORN J* 48:201, Aug 1988.

Steinberg ME: *The hip and its disorders,* Philadelphia, 1991, Churchill Livingstone.

Walker JL and others: Centrifugation of antibiotic impregnated bone cement, *Orthopedics* 11:891, June 1988.

Wasilauski SA and others: Value of continuous passive motion in total knee arthroscopy, *Orthopedics* 13:292, March 1990.

Watson M: *Practical shoulder surgery,* London, 1985, Grune & Stratton.

Whipple TL, Ellis FD: A technique for arthroscopic anterior cruciate ligament repair, *Clin Sports Med* 10:463, July 1991.

Yerys P: Arthroscopic posterior cruciate ligament repair, *Arthroscopy* 7:111, 1991.

8

Traumatic Musculoskeletal Injury

Compression, shearing, and tension forces cause injury to the musculoskeletal system, resulting in fracture, dislocation, sprain, strain, open wounds, or contusion. Injury can be caused by trauma, bone fatigue, or changes in the structure of the bone secondary to osteoporosis or disease, such as a tumor. Immediate threat to the patient's life from an injured extremity is uncommon unless it is associated with injuries of the thoracic, spinal, peritoneal, or cranial cavities. Neurologic and vascular compromise is also a consideration for immediate treatment. Treatment of injuries to other systems may be required before or during orthopaedic treatment. The surgical treatment is determined taking into consideration the length of time for healing, the anticipated postoperative activity level, and any accompanying injury or disease processes. The injury type determines the nursing care to be implemented intraoperatively.

NURSING CARE

Nursing diagnosis will vary depending on the type and severity of the injury and the patient's age, medical history, and surgical history, as well as other factors. Nursing care for a patient with traumatic musculoskeletal injury is consistent with that provided for other patients (see Chapter 4). Caring for a patient with a traumatic injury requires collaboration with other units and disciplines, including the emergency center, the radiology department, the laboratory, and the physician. Communication is a key component of effective collaboration. Nursing personnel should understand the mechanism of the traumatic injury and

have knowledge of the anticipated procedures and necessary equipment. An operating room caring for patients with orthopaedic trauma requires specialized equipment. Initial purchase plans should be discussed with the physicians using the equipment, because few hospitals can purchase multiple systems. A physician must be comfortable with the system being used; if a desired system is not available, product representatives may work with the hospital to provide supplies as needed. In an era of cost containment, it is important to meet patient care needs without overstocking an operating room. Basic instrumentation systems needed to care for patients with traumatic injury include:

- Instrumentation for implants for open reduction or internal fixation of all anatomic sites
  - Plates (dynamic compression plate [DCP]), side plate and screw, supracondylar, buttress) (Fig. 8-1)
  - Screws (stainless steel or titanium matched to the implant being used) (Fig. 8-2)
  - Pins
- Instrumentation for implanting intramedullary rods or nails into the upper and lower extremities (Fig. 8-3)
- Instrumentation for external fixation (Fig. 8-4)
- Instrumentation for spinal fixation
- Pulsatile lavage equipment
- Specialty supplies, such as cable, wire, and reduction clamps, for varied anatomic sites
- Compartment pressure monitor (Fig. 8-5)
- Fracture table, traction bow, and other positioning equipment (Fig. 8-6)

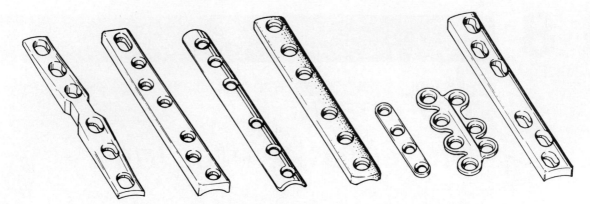

Fig. 8-1   Examples of fixation plates: TOD, plate with compression slot, semitubular, neutralization, small-fragment, DCP. (From Gustilo RB, Kyle RF, Templeman D: *Fractures and dislocations,* vol 1, St Louis, 1993, Mosby.)

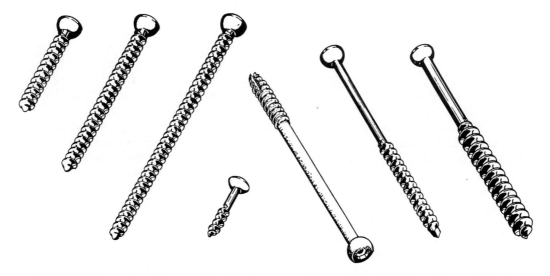

Fig. 8-2   Examples of screws for fixation: cancellous and cortical, lag, pretapped and self-tapping. (From Gustilo RB, Kyle RF, Templeman D: *Fractures and dislocations,* vol 1, St Louis, 1993, Mosby).

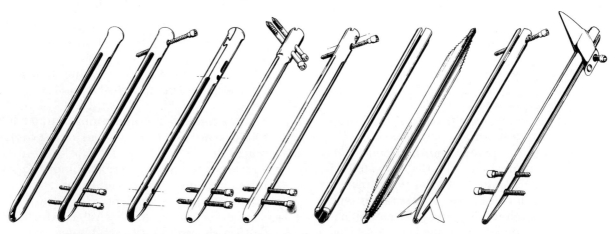

Fig. 8-3   Examples of intramedullary fixation devices: AO, AO or Grosse-Kempf interlocked, AO Universal, Recon, Russeu-Taylor interlocked, Küntscher, Schneider, Brooker-Wells, Williams (Kütscher) Y-Nail. (From Gustilo RB, Kyle RF, Templeman D: *Fractures and dislocations,* vol 1, St Louis, 1993, Mosby.)

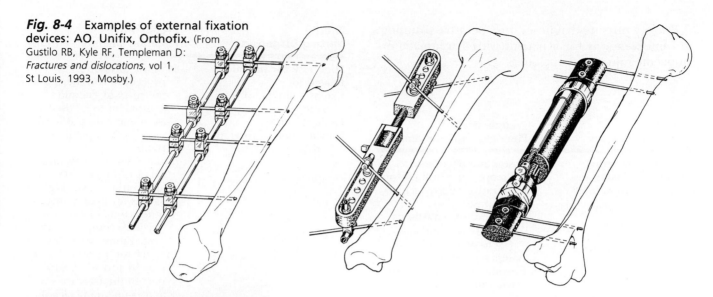

Fig. 8-4 Examples of external fixation devices: AO, Unifix, Orthofix. (From Gustilo RB, Kyle RF, Templeman D: *Fractures and dislocations,* vol 1, St Louis, 1993, Mosby.)

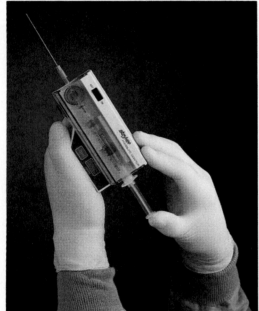

Fig. 8-5 Compartment pressure monitor. (Courtesy Stryker Surgical.)

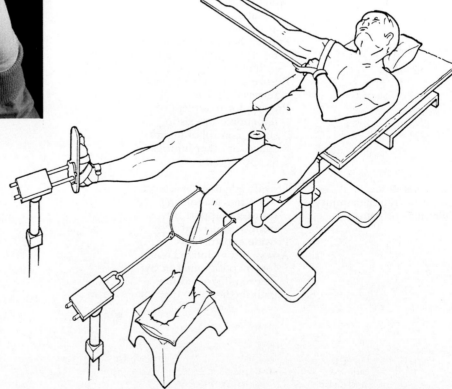

Fig. 8-6 Patient positioned supine on fracture table for intramedullary rodding. (From Gustilo RB, Kyle RF, Templeman D: *Fractures and dislocations,* vol 2, St Louis, 1993, Mosby.)

Priority nursing diagnoses, preoperative planning, and interventions for a patient with a traumatic orthopaedic injury may include:

Priority Nursing Diagnoses	Preoperative Planning and Interventions
Sensory/perceptual alterations related to: Tissue perfusion in affected extremity	Assess and document: Preoperative and postoperative neurovascular status Absence of parasthesia Intact movement and sensation Assess sensory status Provide orientation to surroundings
Altered tissue perfusion related to: Extent of traumatic injury, trauma, and swelling of soft tissue at operative site Use of pneumatic tourniquet Preexisting medical conditions	Assess and document: Peripheral pulses Extremity warmth Capillary refill Apply antiembolic stocking (for high-risk patients) Apply pneumatic tourniquet correctly, verify pressure settings, monitor throughout the procedure, and assess
High risk for fluid volume deficit related to: Extent of traumatic injury Medical history	Ensure availability of blood and fluid replacement supplies Monitor fluid loss per observation and catheterize as needed Prepare laboratory requests for intraoperative monitoring Ensure availability of blood retrieval devices Prepare for treatment of impending or existing shock, control of hemorrhage, or other injuries as appropriate
Pain related to: Extent of traumatic injury Tolerance of pain	Provide adequate assistance when moving, during transfer; support the extremity as needed Provide explanations Assess and maintain comfort by positioning or by determining need for pain medication

Priority Nursing Diagnoses	Preoperative Planning and Interventions
High risk for infection related to: Extent and type of traumatic injury Medical history Implantation of foreign body	Plan the location of the procedure considering the surgical site and equipment to be used so as to maintain traffic patterns in the operating room Cleanse site prior to surgical skin preparation (use appropriate cleansing agents for grease, dirt, or other contamination as needed); complete skin preparation per policy Prepare for an "open" fracture by providing support to the fracture site and maintaining cleanliness Monitor sterility of instrumentation, fixation supplies, and any implants required Prepare antibiotic irrigation Prepare for pulsatile lavage or irrigation as needed Administer preoperative intravenous antibiotics
High risk for altered body temperature related to: Extent and type of traumatic injury	Provide warm blankets preoperatively; use a hyperthermia blanket as needed Minimize patient exposure Organize activities to minimize intraoperative time by planning activities, checking equipment preoperatively, notifying support services such as radiology and laboratory, and preparing equipment to remove temporary stabilizers, such as cast and/or pins Warm solution; control room temperature

Priority Nursing Diagnoses	Preoperative Planning and Interventions
Anxiety and/or fear related to: Extent of traumatic injury Knowledge deficit regarding surgical intervention and outcome	Provide explanations and reassurance to the patient and family Assess need for patient teaching and the patient's readiness to receive information to relieve anxiety Provide information to the family or significant other during the procedure Provide explanations of the anticipated outcome as appropriate Provide opportunities for the family to remain with the patient Assess spiritual needs; offer pastoral or other support as needed
High risk for injury related to: Extent of traumatic injury Acuity level of procedure Surgical positioning required Use of radiography	Continually assess for injury to other systems Ensure that implants and instrumentation are available and that sets are complete Assess competency level of personnel and numbers of support persons available Maintain safety measures during transport and transfer Apply leaded shields to provide protection of sensitive tissue from sources of radiation Check labels carefully (medications, blood, implants) Check equipment function preoperatively; implement safety precautions using equipment Ensure that operative permit is correct

Perioperative nursing practices require continual evaluation and revision of the nursing care plan as care is being provided. The plan of care is implemented, and a postoperative assessment is completed. Many interventions cannot be assessed immediately to determine the long-term outcome; postoperative assessment provides baseline information for evaluating the nursing interventions. Priority postoperative assessment data to gather when caring for a patient undergoing a procedure for trauma includes:

- Neurovascular status
- Skin integrity at sensitive or vulnerable areas:
  - Site of pressure from positioning devices
  - Beneath tourniquet site
  - Preparation site

Documentation of the care provided and the results of evaluation is completed to provide for continuity of care and a record of that care. Documentation on an intraoperative record is individualized for each setting. A summary of the nursing activities impacting the outcome should be reported to postanesthesia care unit personnel. Information that should be documented and communicated following an orthopaedic procedure for trauma includes:

- Implanted devices as appropriate
- Fluid loss and replacement
- Patency of drains; dressings (drainage, bleeding; intactness)
- Precautions and safety measures provided
- Individualized care provided

The text and photographs in this chapter identify techniques implemented during orthopaedic procedures for patients with traumatic injuries. The procedures depict common surgical approaches and select instrumentation. The procedures do not identify each step of the procedure requiring physician consideration but are intended to provide an overview of the procedure to enable the perioperative nurse to anticipate patient care needs. Instrumentation, equipment, and physician preferences change in each setting; therefore it is important to recognize the principles of each procedure and to consider implementation based on an understanding of orthopaedics as a specialty.

■ ■ ■

Orthopaedic perioperative nurses care for patients with fractures of various types and in various locations (see box on pp. 150-151). The basic principles of fracture management apply to most anatomic sites, requiring a basic understanding of the anatomy, the principles of fracture management, and necessary equipment. Three basic goals of fracture management are:

- Reduction or realignment of bone fractures
- Maintenance of realignment
- Restoration of function

Proper names (eponyms) for fractures

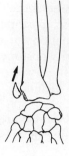

Barton's Fracture
Dorsal rim fracture of the radius

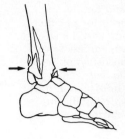

Cotton's Fracture
Trimalleolar ankle fracture of the distal tibia (medial, lateral, and posterior articular margin or posterior malleolus of the tibia)

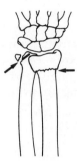

Colles' Fracture
Fractures of the radius and ulna that may or may not involve the wrist joint; caused by extending the outstretched hand

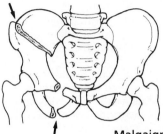

Malgaigne's Fracture
Double fractures in the pelvic ring, causing instability in the pelvis

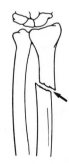

Galeazzi's Fracture
Fracture of the distal third of the radius with associated radioulnar dislocation

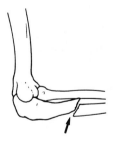

Monteggia's Fracture
Fracture of the shaft of the ulna with displacement of fragments

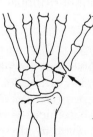

Bennett's Fracture
Fracture at the base of the thumb; acute with associated subluxation or dislocation of the metacarpal joint of the thumb

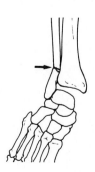

Pott's Fracture
Fracture of the fibula, including malleoli of the ankle

Modified from Mourad LA: *Orthopaedic disorders*, St Louis, 1991, Mosby.

Proper names (eponyms) for fractures—cont'd

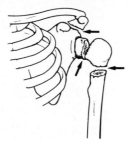

Neer Fracture
Shoulder and humeral displaced fracture resulting in three or more fragments

Salter (or Salter-Harris) Fracture
Fracture may separate the epiphysis from the bone; may involve bones above and below the epiphysis; may be a crush injury to the epiphysis

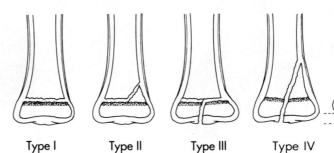

Type I   Type II   Type III   Type IV   Type V

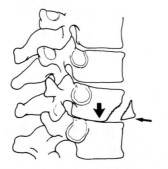

Teardrop Fracture
Compression fracture of the body of a cervical vertebra with separation of a bone fragment

FRACTURE TYPES AND TREATMENT

Fractures are classified as closed or open. Both types can be caused by either a stress injury or pathologic weakening of the bone. Recognizable fracture patterns (Fig. 8-7) include:

Transverse: The fracture is at a right angle to the bone shaft.

Spiral: Bone fragments rotate around one another, resulting in fragmented bone.

Comminuted: Bone is broken into three or more components, each a different size.

Compression: The end of one bone is forced directly into the end of the other

Oblique: Angles of the break or breaks diverge significantly from the perpendicular to the long axis of the bone.

Open fractures penetrate the skin, and the fracture site is exposed, leaving an entrance for microorganisms. Such fractures are considered an emergency and should be reduced within hours of the injury to decrease the chances of infection. Closed fractures are breaks in the bone that do not penetrate the skin.

Treatment of fractures is also classified as open or closed. The decision for treatment is based on the type of fracture and its location and cause. Reduction can be accomplished manually with the application of traction or a cast or by using fixation.

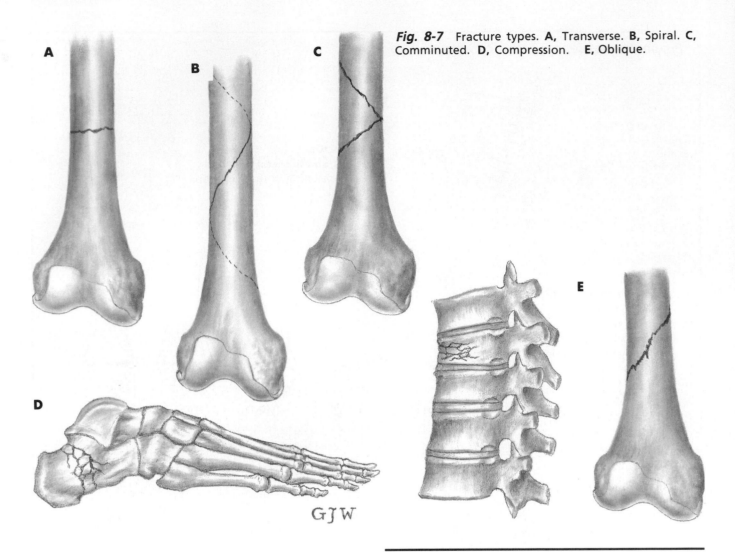

Fig. 8-7 Fracture types. **A,** Transverse. **B,** Spiral. **C,** Comminuted. **D,** Compression. **E,** Oblique.

Closed Reduction

Closed reduction is accomplished by external manipulation of a fracture (following relaxation of the muscles), which forces it into alignment. This eliminates the need to make an incision, resulting in less trauma and potential for infection. The type of fracture must be assessed to determine the possibility of reducing it in a closed manner. Complications that may occur with manual manipulation include increased bleeding into tissue at the fracture site and failure to maintain reduction.

Surgeons may attempt a closed reduction with the patient anesthetized, recognizing that there may be a need to complete the procedure as an open reduction. A fracture may also be managed as a closed reduction followed by an open reduction, internal fixation (ORIF) with surgical exposure to maintain reduction of the fracture for healing.

General procedure for closed reduction

EQUIPMENT AND INSTRUMENTATION ■
Instrument sets and supplies appropriate for the procedure posted
Positioning equipment and other supplies
Drapes if appropriate
Power equipment
Tourniquet
Fluoroscopy or portable x-ray equipment

PROCEDURE ■ A procedure scheduled in the operating room as a closed reduction may require placement of pins or may become an open procedure if the closed reduction fails or reduction cannot be maintained. The perioperative nurse should determine the type of fracture, any previous treatment (a previously reduced fracture where reduction has not been maintained usually results in the need for fixation), and the surgeon's preferences for the type of system to be used to repair the fracture. Preoperative preparation for closed reduction procedures also includes the following:

1 Notify the radiology department of the need for an image intensifier or anteroposterior (AP) and/or lateral x-ray equipment.
2 Obtain necessary supplies and special equipment for a closed reduction with fixation. Obtain positioning equipment, instrumentation, surgical preparation supplies, leaded gowns, and patient protection supplies. Supplies and equipment for an open reduction should be gathered if there is a possibility that the fracture cannot be reduced.
3 Prepare instruments and supplies, including casting materials or a fixation device, for external fixation.

Application of Fixation Devices

Fixation devices can be categorized as external or internal. The objective of fixation is to maintain undisturbed bone healing and restore function.

External fixation is used to minimize surgical exposure. It provides rigid immobilization and can be applied quickly. Types of external fixation include casts, splints, traction, single-bar appliances, and frame appliances.

Cast and splint application

Casts and splints (Figs. 8-8 to 8-11) are external fixators that provide immobilization of a joint or fracture site in order to hold an aligned bone in place until healing takes place. A cast is made of layers of bandages impregnated with either plaster of paris (calcium sulfate) or a synthetic (fiberglass or Thermoplast) stiffener and wrapped circumferentially around the extremity. Splints are used to support a joint or fracture site after reduction has been achieved through internal fixation or closed reduction with pin insertion. Splints are open on one side, and the splint and reduced extremity are wrapped with an elastic bandage to maintain placement of the splint.

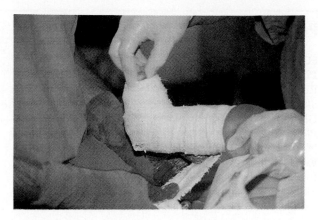

Fig. 8-9 Application of cast material.

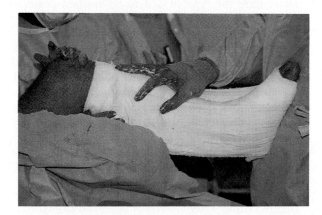

Fig. 8-10 Sugartong splint: protective layer followed by placement of sugartong splint.

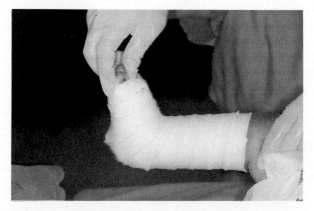

Fig. 8-8 Pediatric lower leg cast: application of protective layer.

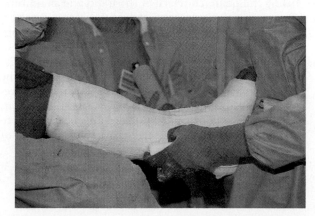

Fig. 8-11 Splint in place before being secured with elastic wrap.

Procedure for cast application

EQUIPMENT ■

Plaster cast
Rolls of plaster
Skin protection—sheet wadding, Webril, or stockinette
Gloves
Plastic-lined pail
Water, cool to lukewarm
Fiberglass cast
Rolls of fiberglass
Skin-protective material for fiberglass casts
Gloves
Pail
Water
Cream or elastic bandage

PROCEDURE ■

1 Determine the type of cast to be applied postoperatively.
2 Obtain casting materials before the procedure is completed. Plaster of paris or knitted fiberglass are two commonly used materials. Plaster of paris should never be opened in the operating room before the incision is closed because the particulate matter that becomes airborne may contaminate the surgical site. Product instructions should be followed for application.
3 Prepare water for immersion. Both casting materials have an exothermic reaction, causing a temperature increase. Tepid water should be used to prevent skin damage and to allow time for the cast to be formed before setting. Excess water is squeezed from the roll.
4 Maintain alignment of the fracture throughout cast application.
5 Wrap the extremity with layers of protective material to protect the patient's skin from the heat of the material used and to prevent cast material from adhering to the skin.
6 Avoid pressure on the cast during application by using the palmar surface of the hand and smoothing to contour the extremity. Allow the cast to set.
7 Elevate the extremity on a pillow or other smooth surface.
8 Check and document the circulation of the extremity before the patient leaves the operating room. The postoperative nurse caring for the patient must receive this information and other communications about the type of injury and treatment in order to adequately assess postoperative complications of casting or bleeding from the surgical site.

> **■ NURSING CARE AND TEACHING CONSIDERATIONS ■**
>
> Drying time is required. A plaster cast should remain uncovererd with the area protected for 48 to 72 hours.
> The extremity should be prevented from becoming wet.
> Range-of-motion and isometric exercises may be appropriate.
> Symptoms to be reported include increased severity of pain, persistent or increased numbness or tingling, less ability to move tissues, burning pain under the cast, and marked edema.

External fixation with appliances

Pin and ring fixators allow stabilization of a fracture at a distance from the fracture site without increasing soft tissue damage. They maintain the length and alignment of a fractured extremity without casting. This allows assessment and treatment of soft tissue wounds, yet permits the patient to resume many activities.

Pin fixators can be subdivided into simple and clamp devices. These allow latitude in pin placement but, following application, do not allow adjustment without replacing the pins. Clamp fixators (or bar appliances) allow for final reduction of the fracture after application of the device, with minor adjustment made by loosening the articulations. These appliances are either single-bar (unilateral) or double-bar (bilateral) devices. The pins are introduced into the cortices of the bone, and the end of each pin protruding from the limb is connected to a bar that runs parallel to the bone. The pin spread and direction of the pins are dictated by the clamp. Simple pin fixator systems are the Roger Anderson device, the Wagner apparatus, the AO frame, the Agee wrist jack, and the Orthofix fixator. Ring fixators allow gradual and precise correction of angulatory and rotational deformity. There is limited access to wounds of the extremity because of the many pieces of the system; therefore tissue transfers may be difficult once the device is applied. Ring fixators include the Ilizarov frame, the Monticelli Spinelli fixator, the Hoffmann fixator and the Ace-Fischer fixator.

Complications of fixation include:
- Pin tract infection
- Pin loosening or breakage
- Limited joint movement
- Neurovascular damage and compartment syndrome
- Malalignment and malunion

The principles for applying any fixator are similar, but an understanding of the specialty instrumentation available for each manufactured device is required.

External fixation of the forearm

DESCRIPTION ▪ Application of an external fixation device.

INDICATIONS ▪ Unstable fracture of the radius.

EQUIPMENT AND INSTRUMENTATION ▪
Soft tissue instruments
Small-bone instruments
Fixation device
Power equipment
Hand table
Tourniquet
Fluoroscopy equipment

PROCEDURE ▪

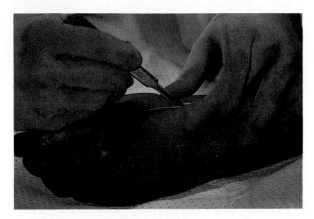

1 The patient is positioned supine with the hand extended on a hand table; a tourniquet is applied to the upper arm, the hand is prepared, and the arm is draped free. A longitudinal incision is made using a No. 15 blade.

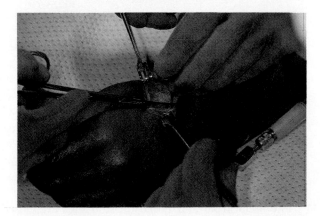

2 Tenotomy scissors are used to dissect soft tissue. Senn rakes are used to retract the incision site.

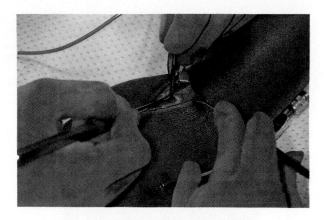

3 A key elevator is used to remove soft tissue from the bone.

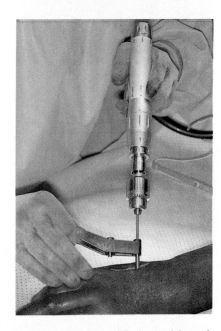

4 The metacarpal drill guide is positioned.

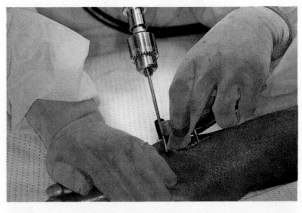

5 The first pin is drilled through the metaphysis of the index and the long finger metacarpal with power equipment.

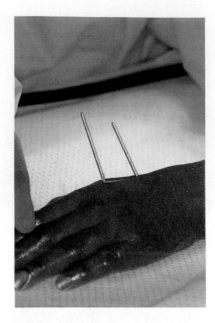

6 The second pin is placed in the index metacarpal shaft.

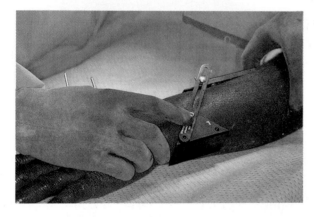

7 The radial shaft pin placement guide is positioned to determine the correct location of the proximal pins. Two vertical lines are marked using a marking pen.

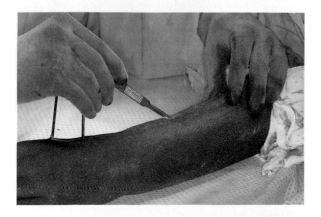

8 A second longitudinal skin incision is made with a No. 15 blade using the pins as a guide.

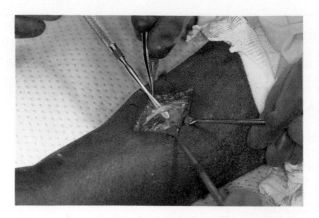

9 The terminal branches of the radial nerve and artery are identified.

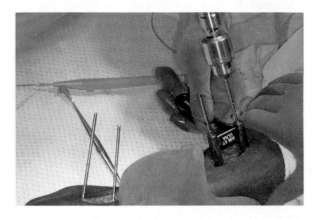

10 The drill guide is placed on the radial shaft, and a pin is drilled through both cortices of the radius. The second pin is inserted in the same manner. Fluoroscopy or x-ray imaging is used to verify the position.

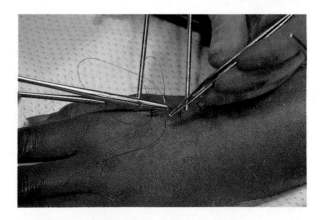

11 The metacarpal and radial incision sites are closed with nonabsorbable sutures.

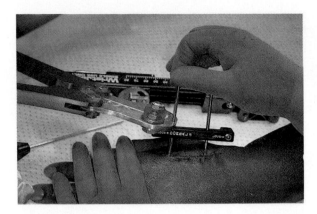

12 The wrist jack is assembled.
   a. The metacarpal bar is applied and tightened, and the pins are cut with a pin cutter.

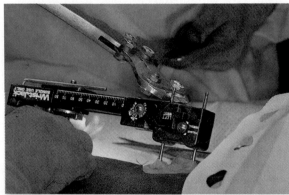

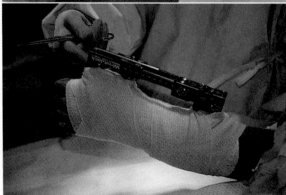

   b. The wrist jack is positioned on the proximal pins; the metacarpal bar is mounted and locked with a screwdriver. The wrist jack is adjusted for fracture reduction. The pins are cut.

13 A soft dressing is applied.

■ NURSING CARE AND TEACHING CONSIDERATIONS ■

Assess the extremity following deflation of the tourniquet.
Encourage immediate ambulation.
Provide patient teaching:
   ■ The pin sites should be cleansed daily with soap and water.
   ■ Symptoms of pin site complications should be reported.

External fixation of the elbow

DESCRIPTION ■ Fixation of bone by placement of an external fixator until healing can take place.

INDICATIONS ■ Need for limb lengthening by epiphyseal distraction or corticotomy, varus/valgus or torsional deformity, nonunion or delayed union, arthrodesis, open (and some closed) fractures, or stiff joints (need for mobilization).

EQUIPMENT AND INSTRUMENTATION ■
Large-bone instruments
Soft tissue instruments
External fixator instruments
Power drill
Tourniquet

PROCEDURE ■

1 The patient is placed in the semilateral position with sandbags beneath the affected shoulder. A tourniquet is placed. Following the incision and soft tissue dissection to the elbow joint, application of the external fixator begins.

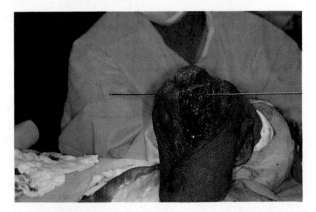

2 A Kirschner wire (1.5 or 2 mm) is used to penetrate the distal humerus in a transverse direction.

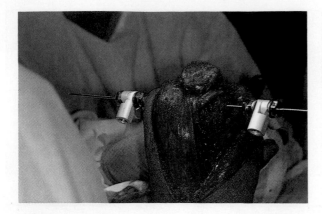

3 Sliding clamps are placed on both ends of the Kirschner wire.

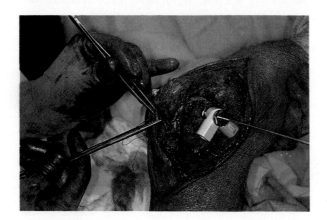

4 The capsule of the elbow is closed with a Maxon suture.

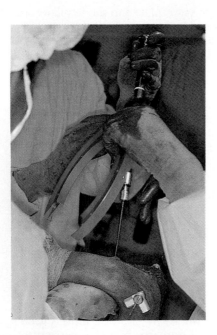

5 A three-quarter ring is placed on the Kirschner wire.

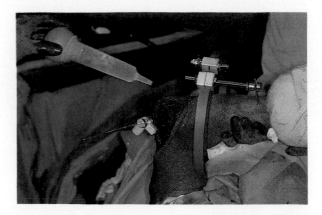

6 Following placement of a second Kirschner wire in the distal end of the radius and ulna, the incision site is irrigated. A third Kirschner wire is placed at an angle in the same area. Columns with sliding clamps for wire holders are placed.

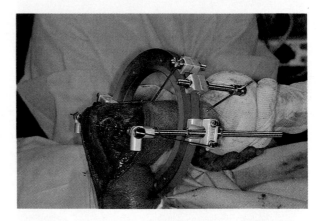

7 A threaded rod is placed between the couplers.

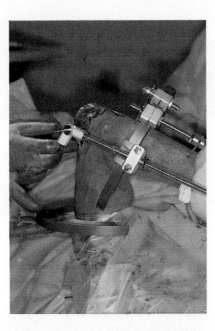

8 The fixation device is built using the second three-quarter ring.

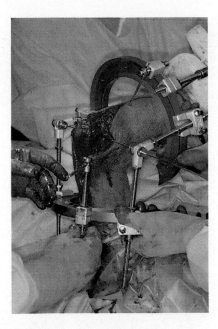

10 A fourth Kirschner wire is placed on the distal end of the humerus. The columns with the sliding clamps for the pin/Kirschner wire holders are placed.

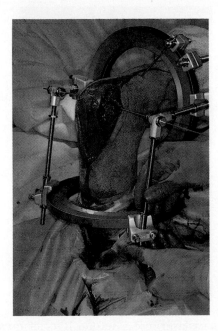

9 Couplers are placed on the ring for rod placement at the proximal end of the humerus.

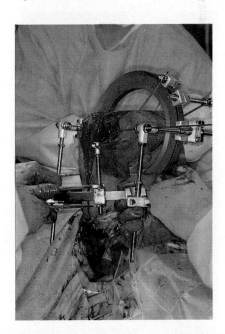

11 The bolts on the threaded rod are lengthened.

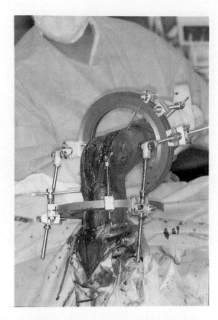

12 One Kirschner wire is removed after the fixation device stabilized.

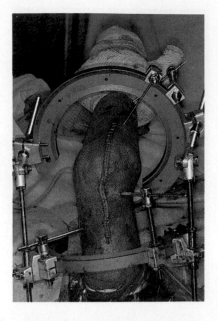

14 Staples are used to approximate the skin.

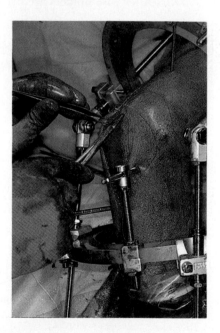

13 The incision site is closed with an absorbable suture.

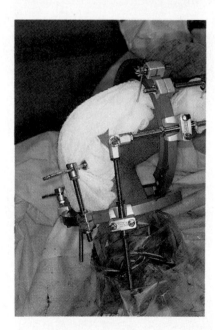

15 A contact layer and a second layer of dressing are applied. Tape and an elastic bandage are applied.

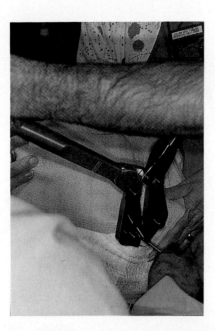

16 The pin cutter is used to decrease pin length.

■ NURSING CARE AND TEACHING CONSIDERATIONS ■

Assess the patient's understanding of the postoperative outcome, including the appearance of the fixator and the patient's ability to manage activities. Determine the patient's understanding of postoperative instructions and ability to follow them.

Ensure protection during positioning; position the affected side near the edge of the bed and assess any potential for injury as the extremity is moved during the procedure.

Postoperatively, assess circulation in the extremity.

Ensure that pin sites are protected during dressing application.

Reinforce pin site care instructions, including cleansing with soap and water.

If the procedure has been done to lengthen a limb, ensure that the patient and family will follow the protocol for the procedure.

Internal fixation

Internal fixation requires a surgical incision to expose and realign the fracture site. More than one type of device may be applied to provide bone stabilization. Devices available for internal fixation include circumferential wire, Kirschner wires, screws, plates, pins, rods (Nails), or nail-and-plate combinations.

Circumferential wire fixation (circlage) (Fig. 8-12) has been replaced for common use by other types of fixation but does serve a purpose in some fractures. It is used for temporary fixation during the plating of long bones, the reattachment of osteotomized greater trochanters, cervical spine stabilization, and for fractures of the olecranon, patella, and medial malleolus. Stainless steel or Vitallium wire, 16 or 18 gauge, is often used. A wire tightener can be used to secure the wire.

Kirschner wires (Fig. 8-13) were originally designed to provide skeletal traction with minimal bone damage but are rarely used for this purpose currently. They are used for fixation in small bones such as those in the hands and feet. A Kirschner wire ranges from 0.7 to 1.1 mm in diameter. Beath pins are Kirschner wires with holes in the end used for passing a suture.

Steinmann pins are also used for fixation in larger bones. The pin sizes range from 1.9 to 2.2 mm in diameter. Steinmann pins can be smooth or threaded.

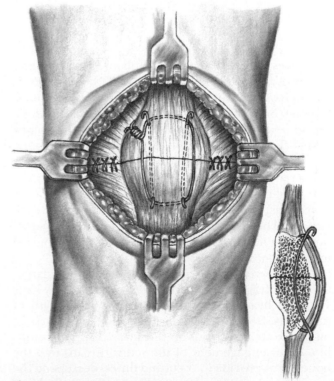

Fig. 8-12 Repair of patella using circlage wire.   GJW

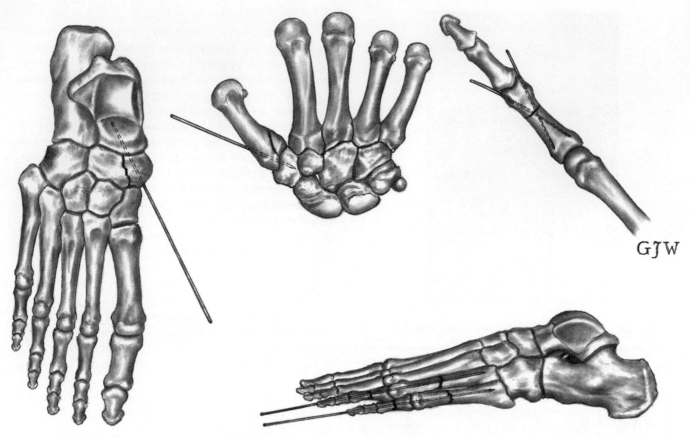

Fig. 8-13   Fixation using Kirschner wire.

Screws are used to attach implants, such as plates and prosthetic devices, to bone; to fix bone to bone; and to fix soft tissues, such as ligaments and tendons, to bone. Screws have different qualities that must be recognized in preparing instrumentation. The screw points (Fig. 8-14) are non-self-tapping, self-tapping, trocar, standard, or pilot point. The holding power of the screw in bone is most dependent on the density and quality of the bone. Bone is either cortical or cancellous, and screws have been developed for each structural need. A Herbert bone screw (Fig. 8-15) does not have a head, so that both screw ends can be buried in the bone. It requires a jig for placement.

Cortical screws are used in diaphyses for both large- and small-fragment or bone plate fixation. They have spherical heads and are threaded the full length of the shafts. Because of its hardness, bone must first be tapped to create threads for the screw. Tapping results in a fuller engagement of the screw threads into the bone. Taps provide four cutting flutes, decreasing the possibility of microfracture and increasing the holding power in the bone.

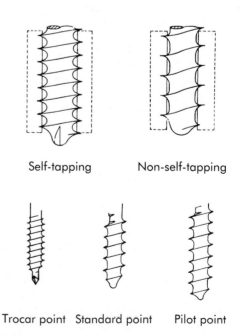

Self-tapping   Non-self-tapping

Trocar point   Standard point   Pilot point

Fig. 8-14   **Screw points.** (Courtesy Zimmer, Inc.)

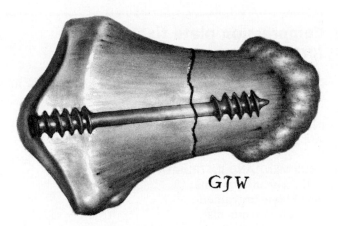

Fig. 8-15 Herbert bone screw for fracture reduction.

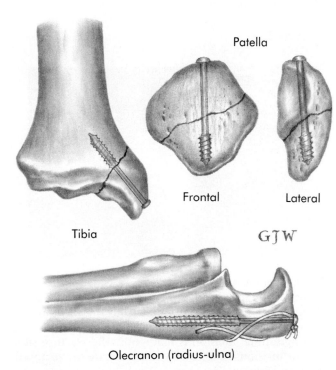

Patella

Frontal   Lateral

Tibia   GJW

Olecranon (radius-ulna)

Fig. 8-16 Cancellous bone screws placed for fracture reduction.

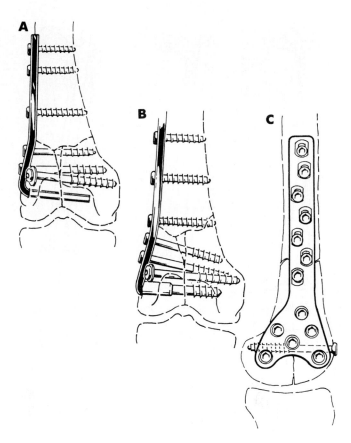

Fig. 8-17 Screw-and-plate fixation devices. **A,** Condylar blade plate. **B,** Dynamic compression screw. **C,** Condylar buttress plate. (From Gustilo RB, Kyle RF, Templeman D: *Fractures and dislocations,* vol 2, St Louis, 1993, Mosby.)

Compared with cortical screws, *cancellous screws* have larger threads with a higher pitch and usually a smaller core diameter (Fig. 8-16). They are only partially threaded. This provides more surface area for contact between screw threads and bone. Cancellous bone is softer; therefore tapping is usually not required unless the screw is being inserted through cortical bone first. Cancellous screws are used in epiphyses and metaphyses for interfragmental fixation.

Plates stabilize the fracture and provide support for bone as it heals. Plates are held in place with screws

(Fig. 8-17) and are available in several configurations and lengths. The plate may be tubular or compression. Use is determined by the location of the fracture, its extent, and the required stabilization. The Swiss Association of Osteosynthesis/Association for the Study of Internal Fixation (AO/ASIF) recommend removal of plates as follows: tibial plates after 1 year, femoral plates after 2 years, and forearm and humeral plates after 1½ to 2 years.

Rods or **nails** are used to stabilize diaphysis fractures of the middle two thirds of long bones. The location of the injury determines the type of rod selected. A rod or nail may be inserted using the closed or open method. As with other systems, instrumentation is specific for the type of rod or nail being inserted (Fig. 8-18).

Nail-and-plates combinations are used for rigid immobilization of the femoral neck when complete prosthetic replacement is not indicated. A nail or lag screw is driven through a slot in the plate, into the femoral head, and through the greater trochanter into the femoral neck. The nail plate is secured to the proximal portion of the femur with screws (Fig. 8-19).

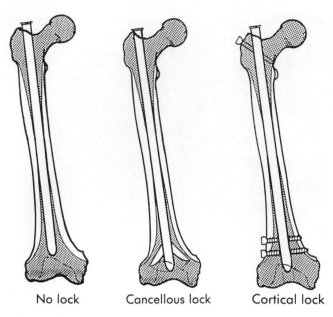

Fig. 8-18 **Nail or rod fixation devices.** (From Gustilo RB, Kyle RF, Templeman D: *Fractures and dislocations,* vol 1, St Louis, 1993, Mosby.)

No lock   Cancellous lock   Cortical lock

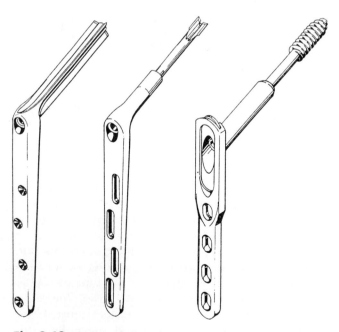

Fig. 8-19 **Nail-and-plate fixation devices.** (From Gustilo RB, Kyle RF, Templeman D: *Fractures and dislocations,* vol 1, St Louis, 1993, Mosby.)

Compression plate fixation of a forearm fracture

DESCRIPTION ■ Application of a plate and screws for internal fixation.

INDICATIONS ■ Displaced fracture of the radial shaft and ulnar shaft.

EQUIPMENT AND INSTRUMENTATION ■
Soft tissue instruments
Small-bone instruments
Fixation instruments
Power equipment
Tourniquet
Hand table
Radiography equipment

PROCEDURE ■

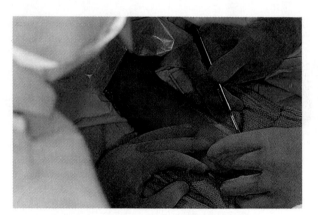

1 The patient is positioned supine with the affected arm extended on a hand table. After a tourniquet is applied, the arm is prepared from the incision site circumferentially. The extremity is draped free. A longitudinal incision is made over the fracture site. The incision is extended to accomodate the required plate length.

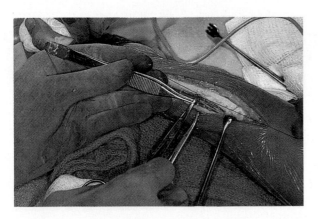

2 Retractors are placed to enhance exposure. Vessels are ligated using a hemostat, Adson forceps, and ties. A cautery can also be used.

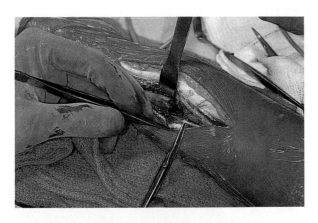

3 The radial nerve is identified and dissected.

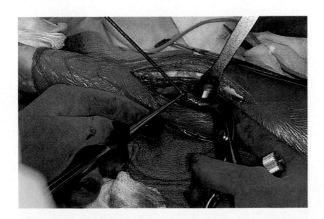

4 Clotted blood and fragments are cleared using a curette.

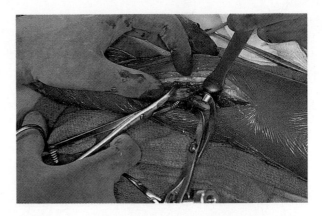

5 Verbugge bone-holding clamps are placed, and the fracture is manually reduced.

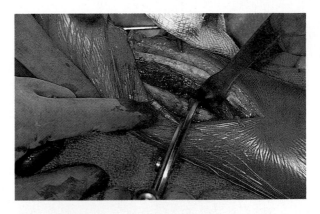

6 Reduction of the fracture site is verified using the image intensifier or x-ray imaging.

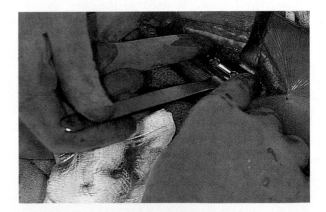

7 The plate is selected.

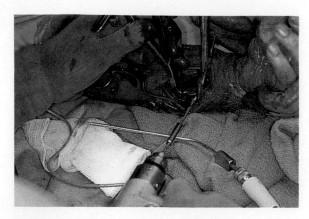

8 Bone-holding clamps are used to secure the plate. Holes are drilled, one at a time, using the power drill and a drill bit.

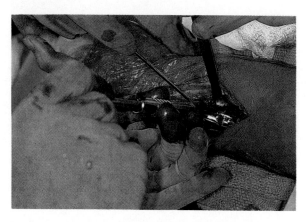

9 The depth gauge is used to measure the screw length. Each screw length is verified by measurement before placement.

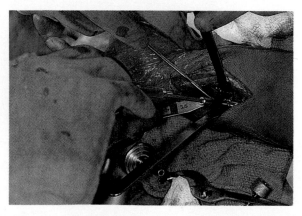

10 The screw hole is tapped to cut the thread in the opposite cortex.

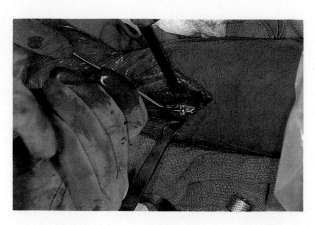

11 Each screw is placed and secured before the next hole is drilled.

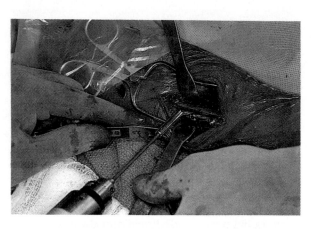

12 Each hole is drilled consecutively, and the procedure is repeated until all screws are placed. Reduction and application of the plate are verified with image intensification or x-ray imaging.

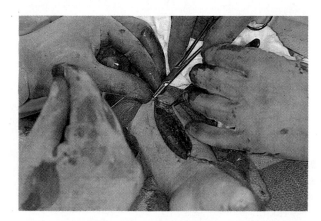

13 The pneumatic tourniquet is released, and bleeding is controlled. Subcutaneous layers are closed with an absorbable suture. The fascia is not closed.

14 The skin is approximated with a nonabsorbable suture.

15 A dressing is applied. A contact layer, an intermediate layer, and Kerlix are used.

16 A sugartong splint is applied on the forearm.

17 An elastic bandage is used to secure the splint.

■ NURSING CARE AND TEACHING CONSIDERATIONS ■

Assess the extremity immediately postoperatively; protect the extremity during transfer, and elevate it immediately postoperatively.

Reinforce preoperative teaching of care of the splint:

- The splint is worn for approximately 6 weeks.
- Activities can be resumed gradually and maintained to a level of comfort.
- The plate can be removed if symptoms of problems develop but not before 18 to 24 months postoperatively.

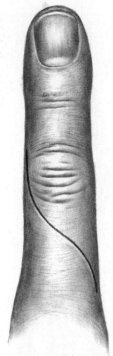

GJW

1 The patient is positioned supine with the arm extended on a hand table. A tourniquet is applied to the upper arm; the skin is prepared from the fingertips to the tourniquet, and the arm is exsanguinated with an elastic bandage. The incision site is marked, and the incision is made with a No. 15 blade.

Open reduction and internal fixation of metacarpal fractures

DESCRIPTION ■ Correction of phalangeal or metacarpal fracture(s).

INDICATIONS ■ **Open reduction:** for unstable fractures or those that are intraarticular or displaced or when closed methods of correction are unsuccessful. **Internal fixation:** for fractures that can be corrected under direct visualization when the wound is irrigated.

EQUIPMENT AND INSTRUMENTATION ■
Small-bone instruments or hand set
Instrumentation for correction of the fracture
Hand table
Tourniquet
Power equipment
Fluoroscopy or x-ray equipment and protective attire

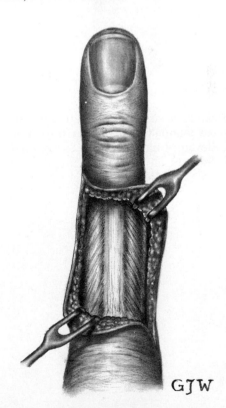

GJW

2 Soft tissue is dissected and retracted with a double skin hook (or Senn Retractor).

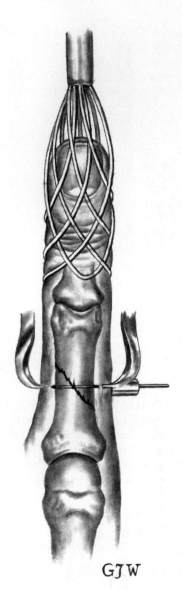

GJW

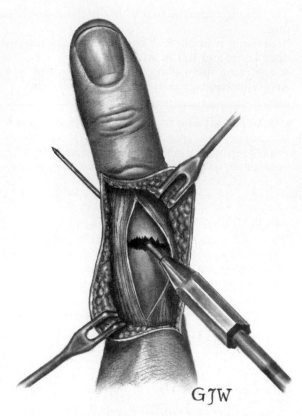

GJW

4 A .035 to .045 Kirschner wire is inserted using power equipment. Correction of a fracture may require insertion of several Kirschner wires, insertion of miniplates, or screw fixation. The method of fixation used to maintain bone lenth and alignment is determined by the surgeon.

3 The fracture is visualized. The fracture site may be distracted manually, or a finger trap(s) may be applied. Elevators may be needed to assist in reduction of the fracture.

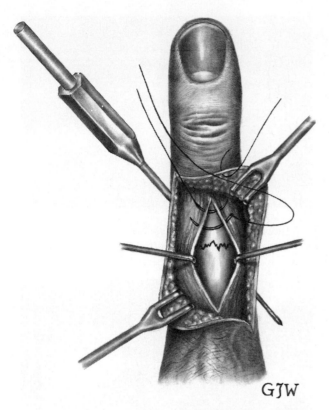

GJW

5 The incision(s) is approximated with a nonabsorbable suture. The pins are cut using a pin cutter. A bulky dressing is applied, and the hand is splinted for support.

■ NURSING CARE AND TEACHING CONSIDERATIONS ■

The length of time required for splinting depends on the type of fracture and the repair technique. Instructions for postoperative pin care, including twice-daily cleansing of the pin site with cotton swabs and hydrogen peroxide are reinforced.

Repair of a patellar fracture

DESCRIPTION ■ Internal fixation for patellar fracture repair. (Fractures of the patella constitute almost 1% of all skeletal injuries occurring from direct or indirect trauma. Opinions differ on the proper treatment, especially in reference to patellectomy. Nonoperative treatment is indicated when fragments are not displaced.) The internal fixation may be carried out using a circumferential wire loop, screws, pins, or a combination of these.

INDICATIONS ■ Fracture of the patella.

EQUIPMENT AND INSTRUMENTATION ■
Large-bone instruments
Soft tissue instruments
Wire tightener
Kirschner wires
18-gauge wire
Tourniquet

PROCEDURE ■

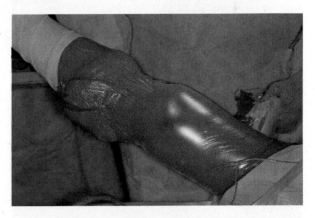

1 The patient is positioned supine on the bed, and a tourniquet is applied to the upper thigh. The surgical site is prepared from the incision to the upper thigh and the lower leg, circumferentially.

2 The leg is draped free; an Ioban-impregnated drape is applied.

3 Following the initial skin incision, soft tissue is dissected using a knife and forceps. Suction is used.

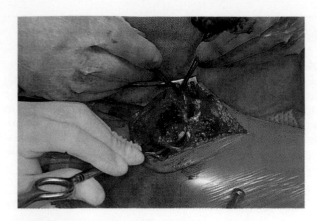

4 A rake retractor and self-retaining (Weitlaner) retractor are placed; blood clots are removed using forceps.

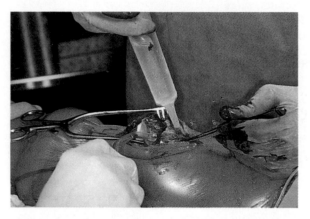

5 The joint is irrigated with normal saline.

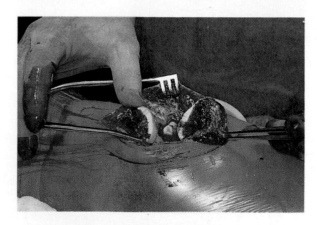

6 The patellar fragments are inspected.

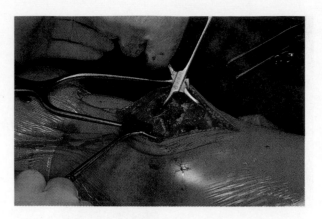

7 A Lewin bone clamp is used to approximate the fragments.

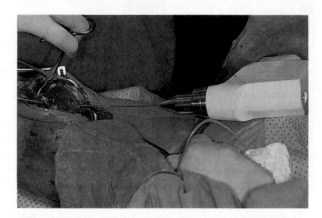

8 A wire driver is used to insert a ³⁄₃₂ Kirschner wire.

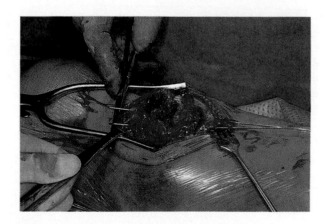

9 A second wire is inserted horizontally.

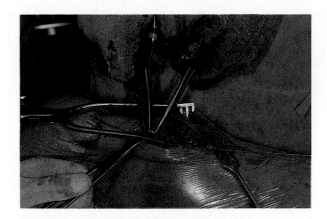

10 A wire twister is used to bend the wires.

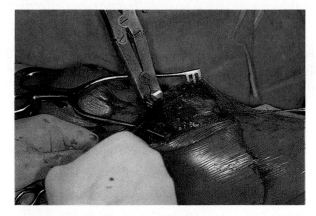

11 The patella is sutured with a heavy, nonabsorbable suture (No. 1 Ethibond).

12 Excess length of wire is cut using a wire cutter.

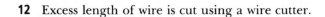
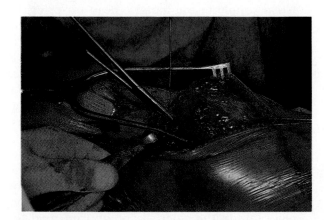

13 The patella is secured using a heavy clamp to pass 18-gauge wire.

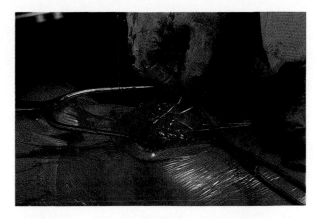

14 The wire is tightened in a circlage manner.

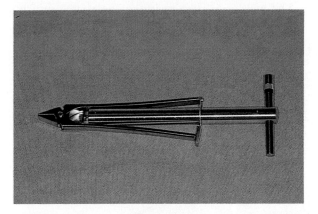

15 A wire tightener is used to twist and tighten the ends of the wire.

16 Using the wire twister, the ends of the wire are bent to lie against the patella.

17 One end of the Kirschner wire is secured flat against the patella.

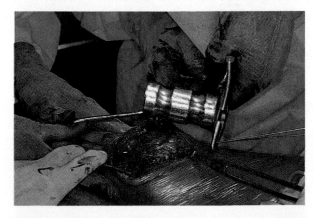

18 The protruding end of the Kirschner wire is held with the wire twister, and a mallet is used to pull the wire secure. The wire cutter is used to cut the wire, and the wire twister is used to secure it against the patella by bending.

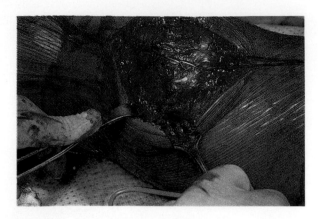

19 The patellar fragments are secured (see Fig. 8-12).

20 The incision is closed with an absorbable suture (2-0 Vicryl).

21 The skin edges are approximated with staples.

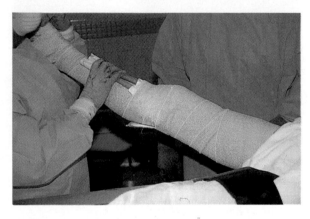

22 Following application of the dressing, hot ice is applied.

23 The leg is wrapped with Kerlix and an elastic bandage, leaving the ends of the hot ice pad protruding.

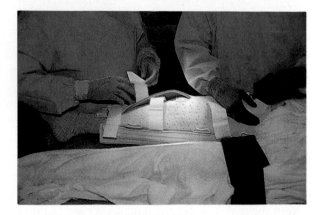

24 A knee immobilizer is applied.

■ NURSING CARE AND TEACHING CONSIDERATIONS ■

Assess other systems for injuries if the injury has resulted from trauma.

Assess the circulatory status of the extremity preoperatively and before the dressing is applied.

Place an adequate layer of intermediate dressing to protect the skin from thermal injury.

Begin quadriceps and leg-lifting exercises immediately postoperatively.

Instruct the patient in ambulation with crutches.

Management of femoral fractures

Perioperative nurses planning care for the orthopaedic patient with a femoral fracture can effectively plan and implement the care based on an understanding of the types of fractures and the most accepted treatments, anatomic considerations, types of available implants, and special equipment and supplies needed for the particular procedure.

Anatomic results following a femoral fracture determine the treatment selected. The goal of clinical management is anatomic realignment of the fracture, enabling the patient to return to the previous level of activity. Types of fractures are femoral neck, intertrochanteric, subtrochanteric, and femoral shaft fractures. Fractures may be subclassified according to the degree of displacement or the extent of the fracture:

Femoral neck fracture: More than 100 kinds of fixation devices may be selected for femoral neck fractures. Management may require internal fixation or prosthetic replacement (Fig. 8-20). The blood supply to the femoral head traverses the neck (Fig. 8-21); therefore disruption of the blood supply can occur with a severe fracture, resulting in necrosis. Garden's classification is commonly used to identify femoral fractures (Fig. 8-22). Treatment is determined not only by the degree of displacement, but also by the patient's physiologic age and any preexisting disease (Fig. 8-23).

Intertrochanteric fracture: Intertrochanteric fractures (Fig. 8-24) make up over 50% of proximal femoral fractures. They are classified as stable or unstable. This type of fracture causes a high mortality rate in the elderly. The implant used for treatment is a sliding nail or screw-and-plate device.

Subtrochanteric fracture: Approximately 10% to 15% of femoral fractures are subtrochanteric, occurring in the proximal one third of the femur (Fig. 8-25). This fracture occurs in a highly stressed area of the femur, resulting in a need for anatomic assessment in order to reach a de-

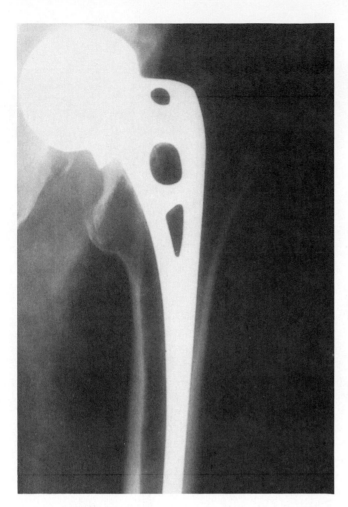

Fig. 8-20 Austin Moore prosthetic replacement for femoral neck fractures. (From Gustilo RB, Kyle RF, Templeman D: *Fractures and dislocations,* vol 2, St Louis, 1993, Mosby.)

Fig. 8-21 Blood supply to femoral head. (From Gustilo RB, Kyle RF, Templeman D: *Fractures and dislocations,* vol 2, St Louis, 1993, Mosby.)

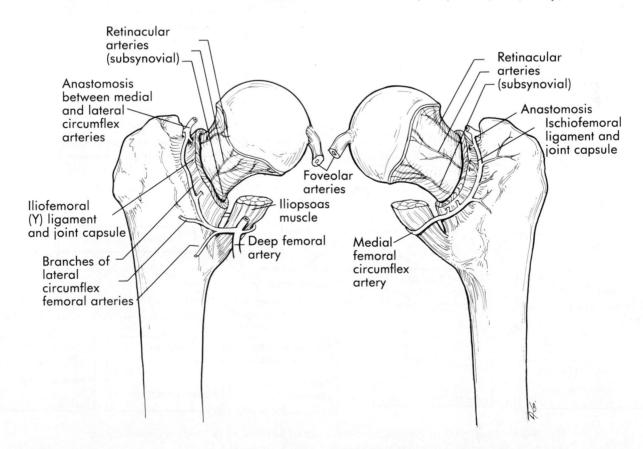

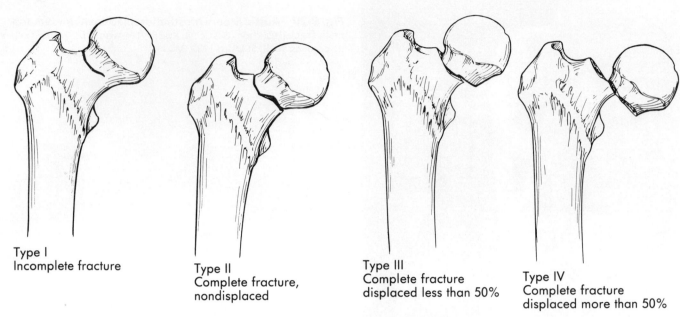

Type I
Incomplete fracture

Type II
Complete fracture,
nondisplaced

Type III
Complete fracture
displaced less than 50%

Type IV
Complete fracture
displaced more than 50%

Fig. 8-22 Garden's classification of femoral neck fractures. (From Gustilo RB, Kyle RF, Templeman D: *Fractures and dislocations*, vol 2, St Louis, 1993, Mosby.)

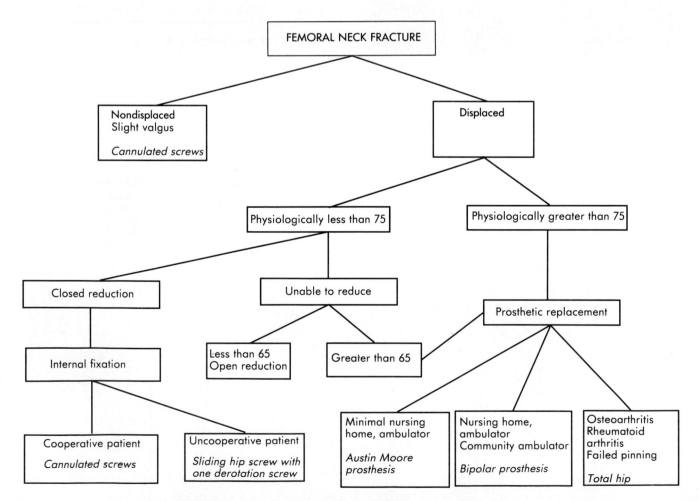

Fig. 8-23 Algorithm of options for treatment of femoral neck fractures. (From Gustilo RB, Kyle RF, Templeman D: *Fractures and dislocations*, vol 2, St Louis, 1993, Mosby.)

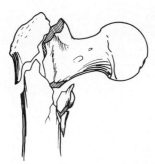

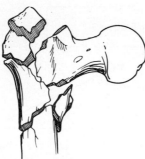
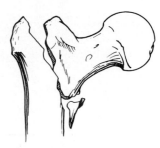
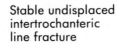

Unstable displaced
fracture of
greater trochanter

Intersubtrochanteric
fracture

Fracture of
greater trochanter

Stable undisplaced
intertrochanteric
line fracture

Stable displaced
intertrochanteric
line fracture

Fracture of
lesser trochanter

Fig. 8-24 **Intertrochanteric fractures.** (From Kyle RF, Gustilo RB, Premer RF: *J Bone Joint Surg* 61A:216, 1979.)

Type I—High   Type II—Low

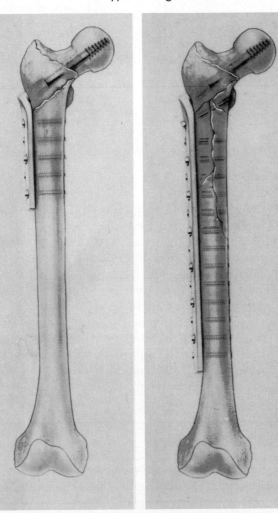
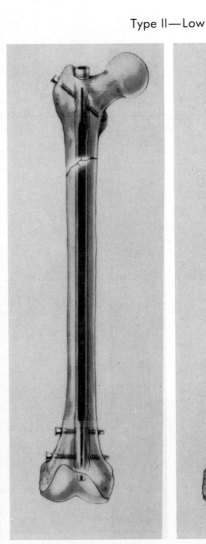
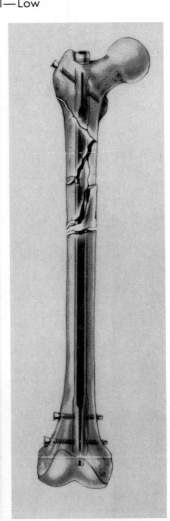

Simple   Comminuted   Simple   Comminuted

Fig. 8-25 **Subtrochanteric fractures.** (From Gustilo RB, Kyle RF, Templeman D: *Fractions and dislocations,* vol 2, St Louis, 1993, Mosby.)

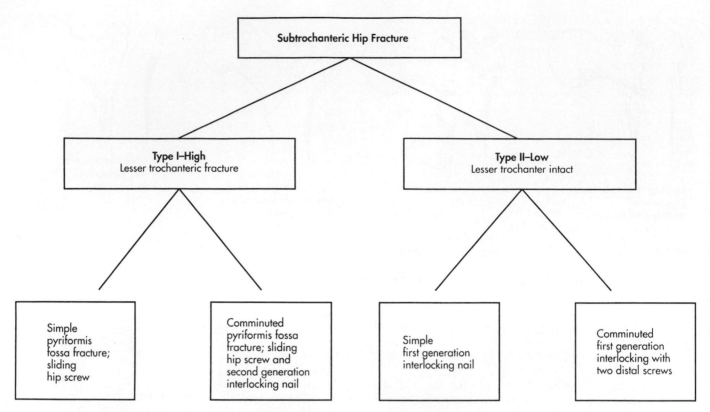

Fig. 8-26 Algorithm of options for treatment of subtrochanteric fractures. (From Gustilo RB, Kyle RF, Templeman D: *Fractures and dislocations,* vol 2, St Louis, 1993, Mosby.)

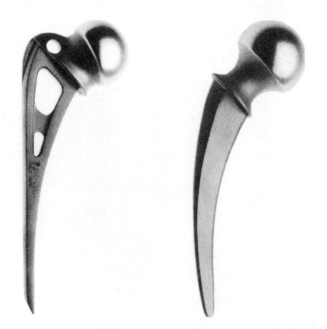

Fig. 8-27 Endoprosthesis for hemiarthroplasty. (Courtesy Zimmer, Inc.)

cision on treatment options (Fig. 8-26). Implants available for treatment are a sliding hip screw device, a first-generation (e.g., a Zickel nail) or second-generation interlocking nail (an intramedullary rod), or a blade plate.

Femoral shaft fractures: Femoral shaft fractures can be classified by location (proximal, middle, or distal) and geometric configuration (spiral, transverse, etc.). The degree of stability is the chief indication for determining treatment, which can include traction, traction and cast bracing, plating, external fixation, and forms of intramedullary nailing.

Hemiarthroplasty

DESCRIPTION ■ Prosthetic replacement of the femoral head (Fig. 8-27) using a single hip component (endoprosthesis). Improved implant design has resulted in three modes of stem fixation: press fit, polymethyl methacrylate (PMMA) cement, and bony ingrowth. (See Total Hip Replacement, Chapter 7.)

INDICATIONS ■ High, displaced subcapital fracture; comminuted, displaced femoral neck fracture; irreducible fracture; severe osteopenia; fracture secondary to neoplasm; associated severe medical problems; nonambulatory patient; or patient with associated neurologic problems, such as dementia, ataxia, hemiplegia, or parkinsonism following traumatic injury.

EQUIPMENT AND INSTRUMENTATION ■
Soft tissue instruments
Large-bone instruments
Instrumentation for the implant
Implant
Positioning supplies
Fluoroscopy or x-ray equipment and protective attire

PROCEDURE ■

1 The patient is placed in a lateral position. The surgical site over the affected hip is prepared and draped. An incision is made using a No. 10 blade, and hemostasis is obtained using electrocautery as dissection is carried through subcutaneous tissue. The self-retaining retractor is placed initially, followed by a hip retractor of choice.
2 The femoral neck and the fracture site are exposed.
3 The femoral head is dislocated and removed with a corkscrew device.
4 The femoral shaft is rasped to accept the selected femoral component.
5 The prosthesis is placed using a bone tamp. Bone fragments are removed using irrigation.
6 The hip is reduced, and an x-ray film is taken.
7 The joint capsule is closed using a nonabsorbable suture. The incision site is closed, and dressings are applied.

■ **NURSING CARE AND TEACHING CONSIDERATIONS** ■

Assess range of motion to attain the correct position during the procedure. Many patients requiring hemiarthroplasty are elderly and therefore may have severe limitations.

Assess for other injuries that may have been caused by the trauma.

Place antiembolic stockings on the unaffected extremity preoperatively and on the affected extremity postoperatively.

Ensure protection and prevention of rotation of the extremity during transfer.

Mobilize elderly and compromised patients as soon as possible postoperatively.

Begin range of motion of the limb immediately postoperatively.

Instruct the patient to ambulate with weight bearing as tolerated beginning at 48 to 72 hours postoperatively.

Multiple pin fixation of a femoral neck fracture

DESCRIPTION ■ Reduction of the fragment and insertion of internal fixation. Steinmann pins, Knowles pins, Hagie pins, and compression screws can all be inserted using the same principles (Fig. 8-28).

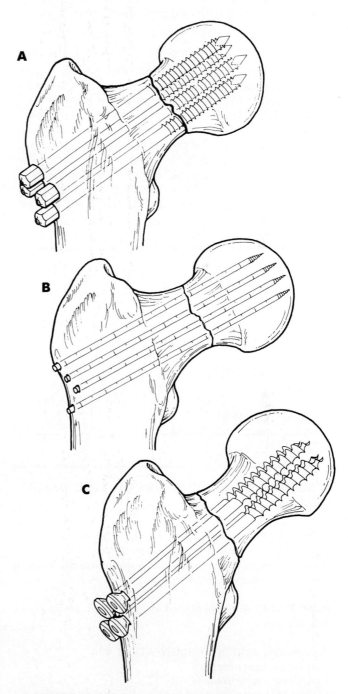

Fig. 8-28 **A,** Knowles pins. **B,** Neufeld pins. **C,** AO cancellous screws. (From McCollister E. *Surgery of the musculoskeletal system,* New York, 1990, Churchill Livingstone.)

INDICATIONS ■ Nondisplaced femoral neck fracture, caused by trauma or disease (metastatic tumor), when closed reduction is not attainable and the patient is not a candidate for hemiarthroplasty.

EQUIPMENT AND INSTRUMENTATION ■
Soft tissue instruments
Large-bone instruments
Appropriate fixation devices
Power equipment
Fluoroscopy equipment and protective attire

PROCEDURE ■

1 Closed reduction is attempted. The patient is positioned laterally on the fracture table with traction on the affected extremity. The patient is prepared and draped. A drape is placed around the hip, and a stockinette is placed over the distal extremity. An incision is made to expose the greater trochanter and the upper femoral shaft area.
2 Fracture surfaces may be irrigated for blood clots. A bone hook is placed on the calcar segment of the proximal neck fragment, and the fracture is anatomically reduced.
3 A guide pin is placed.
4 Fluoroscopy is used to confirm the direction of the guide pin.
5 The pins or screws are placed. The system used determines the number to be placed and the instrumentation required.

■ NURSING CARE AND TEACHING CONSIDERATIONS ■

Crutch walking for ambulation may begin immediately.
Weight bearing is added depending on the stability of the fracture.

Insertion of a compression side plate and screw

DESCRIPTION ■ Correction of a stable or unstable fracture with a screw–and–side plate device. The fracture occurs at an area where blood is supplied to the head of the femur following correction.

INDICATIONS ■ Undisplaced or displaced trochanteric line fracture.

EQUIPMENT AND INSTRUMENTATION ■
Soft tissue instruments
Large-bone instruments
Instrumentation for application of plates and screws
Fracture table
Power equipment
Fluoroscopy or x-ray equipment and protective attire

PROCEDURE ■

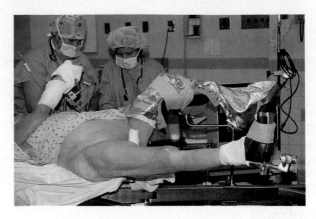

1 The patient is placed on the fracture table in the supine position.

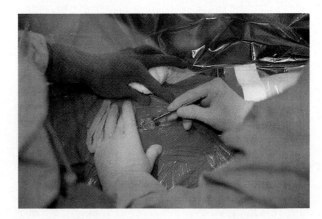

2 The best possible manual reduction is made and confirmed with fluoroscopy. The groin is draped. The operative site is prepared from the waist to the knee, circumferentially. The incision site is draped for exposure.

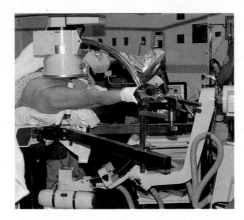

3 A lateral incision is made from the tip of the greater trochanter distally with a No. 10 blade.

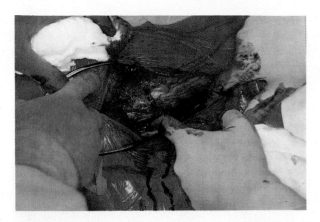

4 The trochanteric region is exposed by sharp dissection through the soft tissue and muscle. A Gelpi retractor is placed.

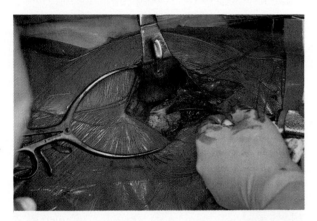

5 Muscle is retracted anteriorly with a Cobra retractor (or a self-retaining retractor). The muscle is incised anterior to the insertion on the linea aspera with electrocautery and elevated subperiosteally from the femoral shaft using a periosteal elevator.

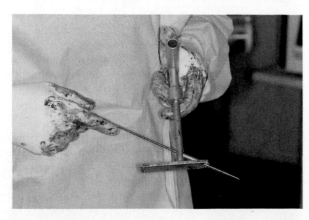

6 A fixed-angled guide is used to pass the guide pin. (A pilot hole may be drilled to establish a track for the guide pin.)

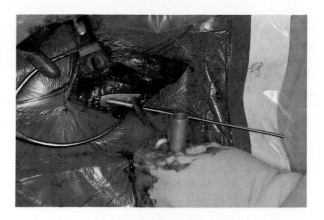

7 The guide pin is driven across the fracture line, in the center of the neck and head of the femur, using the angled guide. Placement of the pin is checked with AP and lateral views.

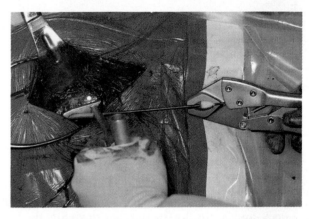

8 Vice-grip pliers are used to change the position of the pin.

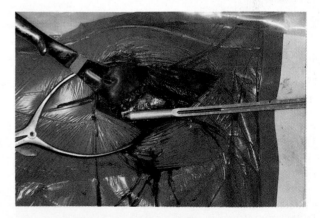

9 A guide pin depth gauge is used to measure the length of the pin inside the femur. The pilot length of the lag screw tap and the reamer depth are determined.

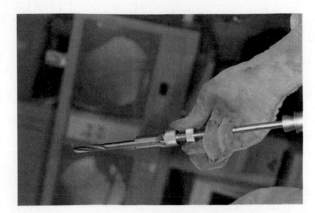

10 A lag screw reamer is assembled.

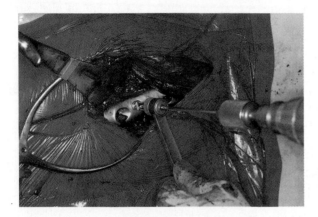

11 The reamer is used to produce a hole in the bone, extending from below the greater trochanter, up the neck, and across the fracture line deep into the head of the femur. The reamer is set at the appropriate length and placed over the guide pin to ream the lag screw channel.

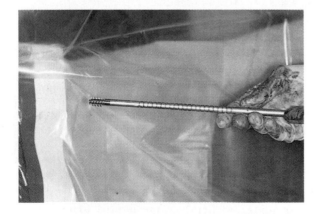

12 A cannulated bone tap is prepared.

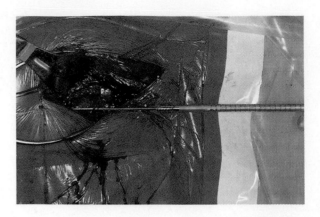

13 With the tap placed over the guide pin, the channel is tapped for lag screw threads. Calibrations on the bone tap are measurements of the distance from the tip of the tap to the rear of the centering collar.

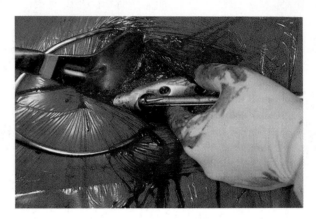

14 The tube plate is placed. Tube plate trials may be used to check the angle of fixation and implant fit. A lag screw of appropriate length and the tube plate are assembled and introduced through the lag screw channel using a T-handle lag screw inserter.

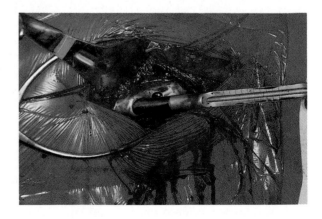

15 The plate impactor is used to seat the plate.

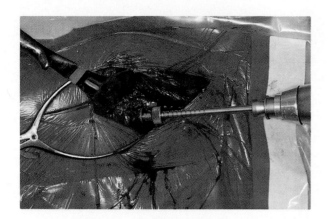

16 The side plate is secured to the femoral shaft using bone screws:

   a The drill bit is introduced using the drill guide. The depth gauge is used to measure screw length.

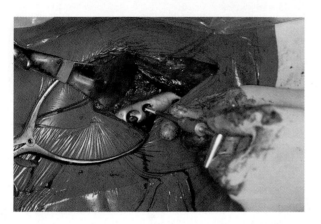

   b The tap is used to prepare the hole for the bone screw.

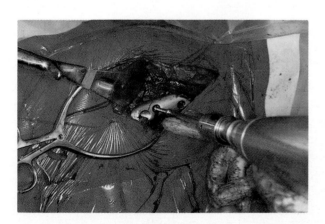

   c Bone screws are placed the length of the plate, repeating each step.

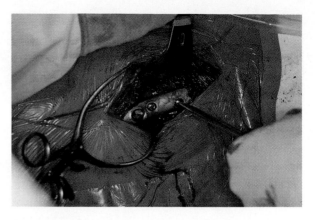

   d The bone screws are secured using a hand-held screwdriver.

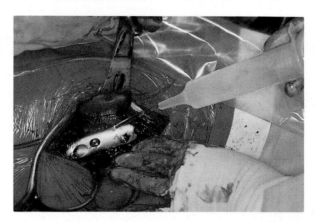

   e A compression screw may be inserted through the lag screw to achieve further impaction and ensure overlap of the lag screw. Placement is verified with fluoroscopy or x-ray imaging.

17 The incision is irrigated.

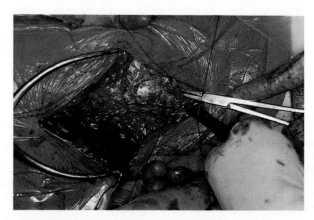

18 A wound drain is placed, and the muscle, fascia, and subcutaneous layers of the incision are closed using a nonabsorbable suture.

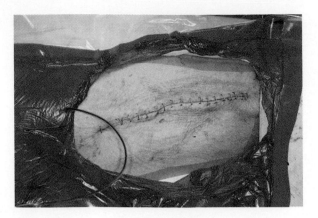

19 The skin is approximated with skin staples. A pressure dressing is applied.

■ NURSING CARE AND TEACHING CONSIDERATIONS ■

Ensure protection of the extremity during transfer.
Assess range of motion to ensure adequate positioning.
Secure and pad the patient on the fracture table.
Instruct the patient about ambulation:
- Ambulation is started 1 to 2 days postoperatively with parallel bars and weight bearing as tolerated; partial weight bearing is begun at the time of ambulation using crutches followed by a walker.
- Full weight bearing is begun at approximately the eighth postoperative week.

Intramedullary rodding of the femur

DESCRIPTION ■ Placement of an intramedullary rod fixation device for alignment of bone.

INDICATIONS ■ Femoral shaft fracture from the lesser trochanter to the lateral epicondyle; pathologic fracture; nonunion; or following osteotomy.

EQUIPMENT AND INSTRUMENTATION ■
Large-bone instruments
Soft tissue instruments
Instrumentation for fixation
Fracture table
Fluoroscopy equipment and protective attire

PROCEDURE ■

1 The patient is positioned supine on the fracture table. The fracture is manually reduced to accomplish anatomic alignment, and alignment is confirmed using fluoroscopy. A pole is placed above the surgical field for securing the occlusion drape.

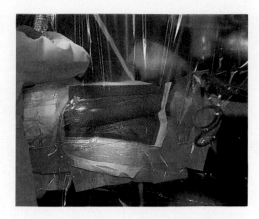

2 The incision site is prepared from the iliac crest to the knee and draped.

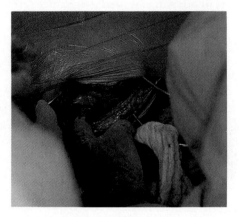

3 An incision is made to expose the greater trochanter. Sharp and blunt dissection is carried out, using self-retaining retractors (Gelpi) to expose the surgical site.

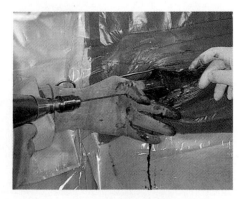

4 A guide pin is driven into the proximal head of the femur using a power drill.

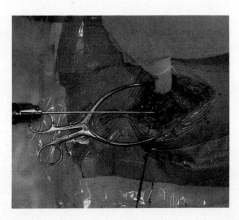

5 The guide wire is advanced to the distal position, and its position is verified with fluoroscopy.

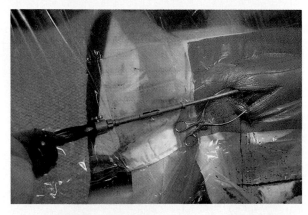

6 Rod length is measured using the measuring sleeve of the fracture reduction tool.

7 The medullary canal is reamed using reamers of graduated sizes.

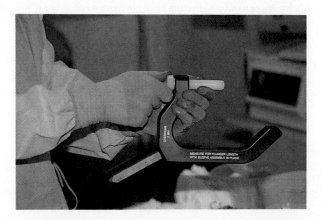

8 The rod connector targeting guide with the proximal femoral plug (white) is assembled.

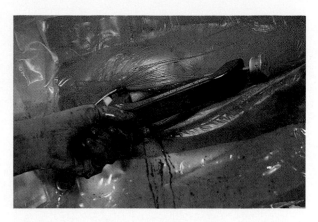

9 The rod connector targeting guide is placed. (Not shown: using the power drill in reverse, the guide pin is removed.)

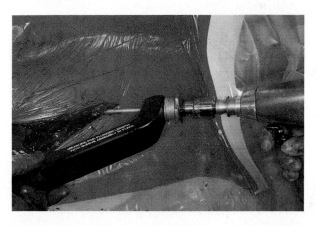

10 The power drill with a drill bit is used to open the lateral cortex of the femoral head. The guide pin will be replaced.

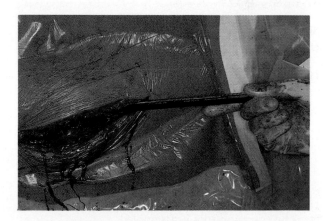

11 A plunger depth gauge is used to measure the length of the lag screw.

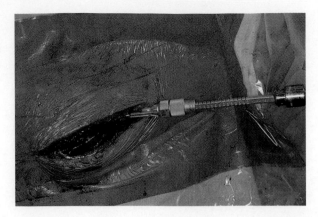

12 A reamer is placed over the guide pin, and reaming is completed until the stop on the device abuts the lateral cortex.

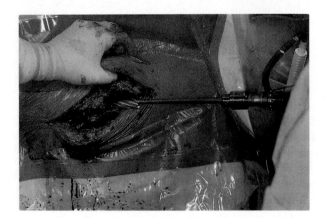

13 Preparation of the femur is completed, using the reamer, to accommodate the rod connector.

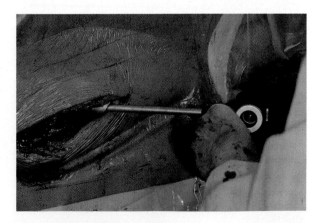

14 The insertion tool is assembled.

15 The lag screw is advanced to the lateral cortex. The insertion tool is removed. A smooth guide wire is also inserted using the rod connector.

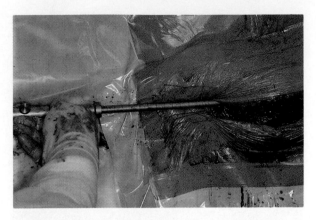

16 The fracture reduction tool is used to maintain alignment of the fracture. The fracture reduction tool is removed.

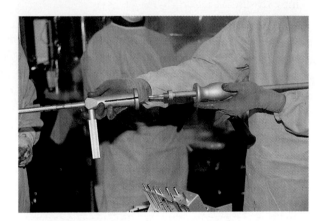

17 An intramedullary rod of appropriate size is attached to the rod driver over the guide wire and tightened with the T-handle wrench.

18 A rotation control handle is attached.

19 The slide hammer assembly is placed on the proximal end of the rod driver.

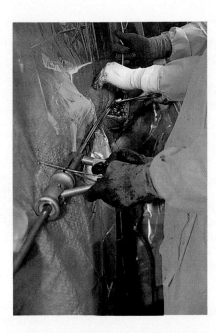

20 The rod is placed over the guide wire and driven into the intramedullary canal. A Kocher clamp is used to deflect the intramedullary guide pin.

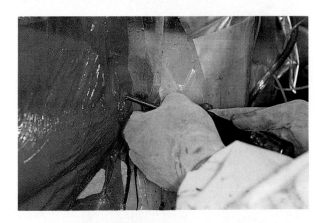

21 Following rod placement, two holes are drilled and screws are selected.

22 Bicortical cross-locking screws are placed, and fluoroscopy is used to verify their placement.

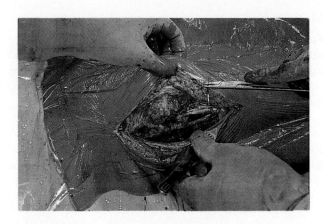

23 The incision site is closed using a heavy suture.

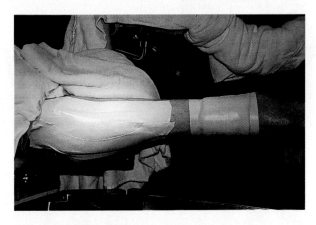

24 A compression dressing is placed.

■ NURSING CARE AND TEACHING CONSIDERATIONS ■

Protect the extremity during transfer.

Assess for injuries of other systems that may have resulted from trauma.

Postoperatively, allow the pain and swelling to subside before beginning quadriceps and knee-bending exercises (approximately 24 hours postoperatively).

Partial weight bearing on crutches with toe touch only is started within several days and maintained for up to 6 weeks or until callous formation begins.

Management of tibial plateau fractures

Vertical loading on the tibial plateau may occur, resulting in fracture. Fractures may be cleavage, medial condyle, or bicondyle, or may be associated with tibial metaphysis and diaphysis. These fracture types are split, depressed, mixed, and bicondylar (Fig. 8-29).

Displaced fractures are treated with open reduction, internal fixation (ORIF). Fixation is accomplished using cancellous screws, Kirschner wire, or buttress plate(s). The fracture pattern, the presence of arthritic changes, osteopenia, or other pathologic involvement will dictate other types of management.

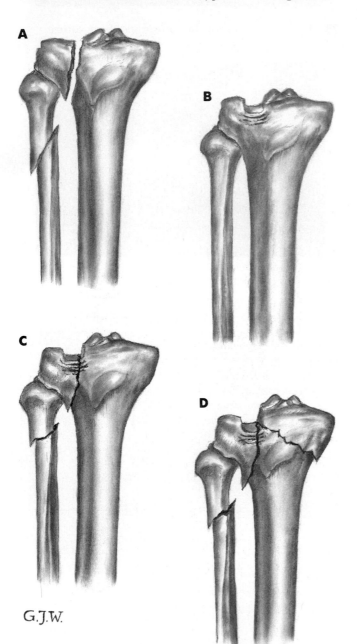

Fig. 8-29 Classification of tibial plateau fractures. **A,** Split. **B,** Depressed. **C,** Mixed. **D,** Bicondylar.

Fixation of cleavage and depressed fractures

EQUIPMENT AND INSTRUMENTATION ■
Large-bone instruments
Soft tissue instruments
Fixation devices (Kirschner wires, plates, screws)
Tourniquet
Power equipment
Fluoroscopy equipment with protective attire

Preoperative preparation
PROCEDURE ■ The patient is positioned supine. Following placement of the tourniquet, the extremity is prepared and draped. Exposure is obtained by making an incision appropriate for the repair.

Fixation of a cleavage fracture
PROCEDURE ■

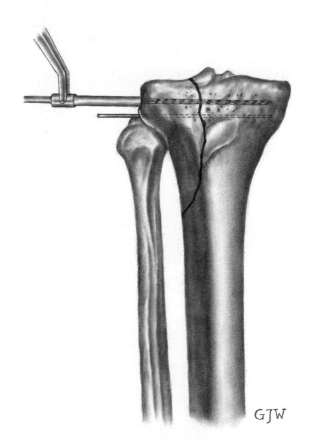

1 A Kirschner wire is placed to secure the fragment. A 3.2 mm drill bit is used to penetrate the cortex, using the drill guide.

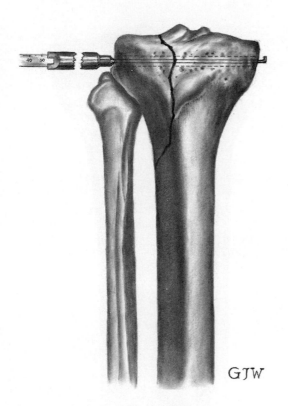

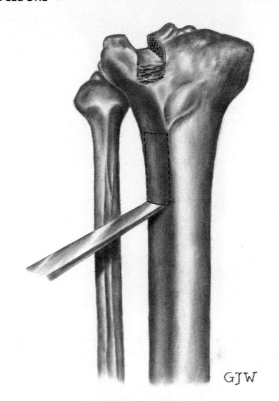

2 A depth gauge is used to measure the tapped cortex.

1 An osteotome is used to prepare a bone flap, below the depression.

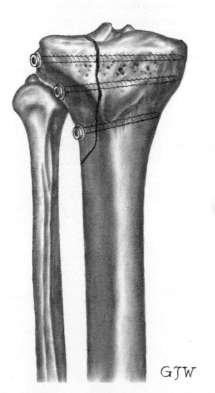

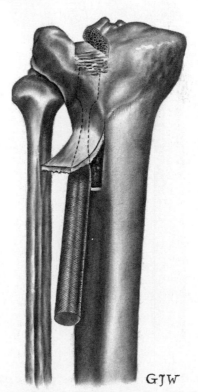

3 Three screws are placed to secure the fragment. Following radiographs for placement verification, the incision site is closed with an absorbable suture.

2 A punch is placed beneath the flap, and the depression is elevated.

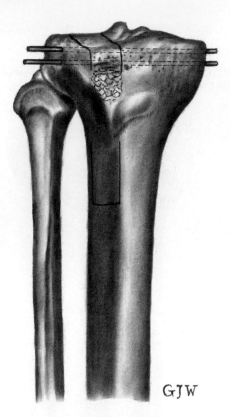

GJW

3 Kirschner wires are placed using power equipment. Radiography is used to ensure reconstruction.

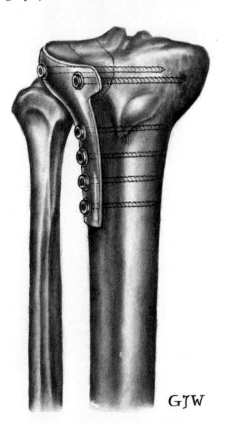

GJW

4 A buttress plate is applied. Cancellous screws are placed in the condyle; cortical screws are placed using a 3.2 mm drill bit, a depth gauge, a 4.5 mm tap, and a screw of the appropriate length. The incision site is closed after the security of the plate has been determined.

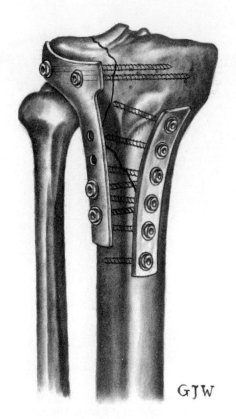

GJW

Severe fractures are treated using multiple buttress plates and screws. A posterior fragment and intercondylar fragment are secured with screws.

■ NURSING CARE AND TEACHING CONSIDERATIONS ■
Protect the extremity during transfer. Maintain movement using continuous passive motion. Restrict weight bearing for up to 10 weeks.

BIBLIOGRAPHY

Association of Operating Room Nurses, Inc.: *AORN standards and recommended practices for perioperative nursing—1992,* Denver, 1992, AORN.

Barrett J, Bryant BH: Fractures: types, treatment, perioperative implications, *AORN J* 52:350, Aug 1990.

Browner B and others: *Skeletal trauma, fractures, dislocations and ligamentous injuries,* vols 1 and 2, Philadelphia, 1992, WB Saunders.

Chapman MW: *Operative orthopedics,* vols 1 and 2, Philadelphia, 1988, JB Lippincott.

Crenshaw AH: *Campbell's operative orthopaedics,* vol 2, ed 8, St Louis, 1992, Mosby.

Freeman MCR, Flanagan ME, Champion HR: Perioperative nursing care of the multiple trauma patient, *AORN J* 50:40, July 1989.

Good LP: Compartment syndrome: a closer look at etiology, treatment, *AORN J* 56:904, Nov 1992.

Gustillo R, Kyle R, Templeman D: *Fractures and dislocations,* vol 2, St Louis, 1993, Mosby.

Hampel G: Closed interlocking nailing in the lower extremity: indications and positioning, *AORN J* 47:1203, May 1988.

Hansell MJ: Fractures and the healing process, *Orthop Nurs* 7:43, Jan/Feb 1988.

Laurin C, Riley LH, Roy-Camille R: *Atlas of orthopaedic surgery,* St Louis, 1992, Mosby.

Meeker M, Rothrock J: *Alexander's care of the patient in surgery,* ed 9, St Louis, 1991, Mosby.

Meyers MH: *Fractures of the hip,* St Louis, 1985, Mosby.

Mourad L: *Orthopaedic disorders,* St Louis, 1991, Mosby.

Rockwood CA, Green DP, Bucholz RW: *Rockwood and Green's fractures in adults,* ed 3, Philadelphia, 1991, JB Lippincott.

Rothrock J: *Perioperative nursing care planning,* St Louis, 1990, Mosby.

Trauma Nursing Coalition: *Nursing care of the trauma patient,* 1992, Trauma Nursing Coalition.

Zuckerman JD: *Comprehensive care of orthopaedic injuries in the elderly,* Baltimore, 1990, Urban & Schwarzenberg.

9

Congenital Anomalies

Congenital anomalies are abnormalities of development present at the time of birth, resulting from an abnormal genetic constitution, from environmental factors, or from a combination of both. Some are readily noticed, requiring correction soon after birth, whereas others may go undetected or not require treatment until later in life. Surgical nurses therefore care for patients of all age groups who require correction of a congenital abnormality. Some disorders are treated nonsurgically; surgical intervention is indicated when the problems cannot otherwise be resolved. Other disorders are treated when the disfigurement or deformity causes pain or interferes with the function of other systems. Anomalies can affect any area of the musculoskeletal system. Children differ from adults in musculoskeletal characteristics and potential for growth. Surgical interventions to correct congenital anomalies of the skeletal system require a plan of care addressing multisystem needs, an understanding of human growth and development, and the evaluative criteria for different age groups.

NURSING CARE

Nursing diagnoses will vary depending on the type of anomaly and the patient's age, medical history, and surgical history, as well as parental support and other factors. Priority nursing diagnoses and interventions provided for a patient with a musculoskeletal anomaly may include those for multiple age groups. Specific diagnoses for an adult are identified in Chapter 7.

Priority Nursing Diagnoses	Preoperative Planning and Interventions
Anxiety and/or fear related to: Parental perception of the cause, surgical outcome Financial impact Parent-child separation Risk of impaired growth and development, pain, disfigurement Discharge requirements Knowledge deficit regarding planned surgical intervention and outcome, discharge instructions	Determine need for reassurance and time to express feelings about the surgical procedure Assess physical and psychologic preparation for surgery Assess parent-child bonding process Assist in management of anxiety and stress by providing opportunities for the family to remain with the patient Answer questions and offer explanations; offer information throughout the surgical procedure; determine alternate methods of allowing children to express feelings Provide spiritual or pastoral support as needed
Altered tissue perfusion related to: Multisystem involvement Ineffective ventilation Limited diaphragmatic excursion	Assess and document respiratory, cardiovascular, and neurologic status Anticipate the patient's specific needs Recognize evaluative criteria for all age groups

Priority Nursing Diagnoses	Preoperative Planning and Interventions
High risk for fluid volume deficit or excess related to: Increased susceptibility for development of fluid imbalances	Ensure availability of blood and fluid replacement Monitor fluid and/or blood loss per observation; catheterize as needed; weigh sponges Prepare laboratory requests for intraoperative monitoring
High risk for infection related to: Use of implanted devices Surgical intervention involving bone	Implement AORN-recommended practices Monitor sterility of implants Administer antibiotics per order
High risk for altered body temperature related to: Body surface area of infants and children Administration of anesthetic medications	Provide warm blankets preoperatively; use a hyperthermia blanket or reflective blankets Minimize patient exposure Organize activities to minimize intraoperative time by having correct-size instruments, special equipment available Warm solutions Increase room temperature for a period of time before the patient enters the room
Impaired physical mobility related to: Congenital abnormality	Evaluate mobility and range of motion Provide assistance during transfer, movement Prepare for positioning by obtaining positioning devices of the appropriate type and size
Body image disturbance related to: Physical abnormality	Discuss anticipated outcome with the patient and family
Pain related to: Degree of involvement requiring surgical intervention	Determine measures to prevent or alleviate pain that can be implemented preoperatively and intraoperatively Provide adequate assistance when moving, during transfer Provide explanations Assess and maintain comfort

Perioperative nursing practices require continual evaluation and revision of the nursing care plan as care is being provided. The plan of care is implemented, and a postoperative assessment is completed.

Many interventions cannot be assessed immediately to determine the long-term outcome; postoperative assessment provides baseline information for evaluating the nursing interventions. Priority postoperative assessment data to gather when caring for a patient with a congenital musculoskeletal disorder include readiness for discharge, understanding of instructions for medication therapy, awareness of postoperative physician appointments, understanding of the signs and symptoms to be reported, and understanding of instructions and the need for physical therapy.

Documentation of the care provided and the results of evaluation is completed to provide for continuity of care and a record of that care. Documentation on an intraoperative record is individualized for each setting. A summary of the nursing activities impacting the outcome should be reported to the postanesthesia care unit personnel. Information that should be documented and communicated following an orthopaedic procedure varies with the many types of procedures completed for congenital anomalies. The report that is necessary may change in an outpatient versus an inpatient setting, based on the amount of teaching acquired preoperatively and the services available to the patient. Priority information may include:

- Preoperative range of motion and limitations and associated pain
- Parent-child psychologic needs
- Preoperative neurologic, respiratory, and cardiovascular status
- Implanted devices as appropriate
- Patency of drains; dressings (drainage, bleeding; intactness)
- Precautions required for positioning
- Fluid loss and replacement
- Preoperative teaching and level of comprehension of parents and child
- Discharge instructions provided
- Individualized care provided

The text and photographs in this chapter identify techniques implemented during orthopaedic procedures for patients with congenital anomalies. Many procedures for correction of congenital anomalies require application of a basic understanding of the anatomy, the correction desired, and implant availability. More important, the surgical nurse must apply principles appropriate for the particular age group based on an understanding of human growth and development.

The procedures depict common surgical approaches and select instrumentation. The procedures do not identify each step of the procedure requiring physician consideration but are intended to provide an overview of the procedure to enable the perioperative nurse to anticipate patient care needs. These procedures can also be implemented for traumatic injuries in the event that a similar course of treatment is considered. Instrumentation, equipment, and physician preferences change in each setting; therefore it is important to recognize the principles of each procedure and to consider implementation based on an understanding of orthopaedics as a specialty.

PROCEDURES FOR COMMON ANOMALIES

The procedures described here include correction of talipes equinovarus (clubfoot), the Ilizarov method for treatment of bone defects, correction of a congenital hip disorder, and tibial osteotomy for limb realignment.

Talipes equinovarus is a common congenital anomaly, occurring in 1 to 3 cases per 1000 live births; it occurs twice as frequently in males. The cause is controversial. Theories include genetic and chromosomal variations with hereditary correlations, intrauterine position or compression of developing tissues, interruption of development during the first trimester, and maternal use of some medications, such as abortifacients and drugs containing curare. Corrective manipulation and casting is used in infants up to 6 weeks of age, followed by manipulation and casting every other week until a surgical procedure is deemed necessary. This is found to be 50% effective as a treatment.

Treatment of bone defects using the Ilizarov method applies the tension-stress principles using gradual controlled distraction of the bone ends to stimulate bone production and support new growth of surrounding tissues. The method is based on the concept that the size and shape of a bone are influenced by the load applied to it and by blood supply. The new tissues grow along the same lines as the distraction force vector. The fixator permits three-dimensional corrections, including rotation, angulation, manipulation of length, and translation. The fixator can be assembled in more than 600 configurations (Fig. 9-1).

Procedures for correction of a congenital hip disorder include closed or open reduction, osteotomy, adductor tenotomy, and arthroplasty. The condition ranges from minimum instability or congruence of the femoral head with the acetabulum to irreducible femoral head dislocation (Fig. 9-2).

Developmental or congenital deformities of the lower extremity or traumatic injury may require a tibial osteotomy. Hyperextension deformities generally occur after trauma that causes closure of the anterior portion of the proximal physis. The osteotomy may be performed in the area of the knee joint, in the midshaft of the tibia, or in the distal tibia.

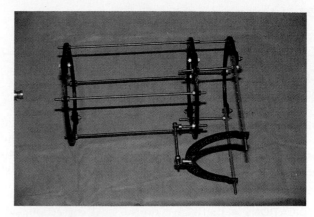

Fig. 9-1 Ilizarov external fixator prepared for placement on the lower extremity.

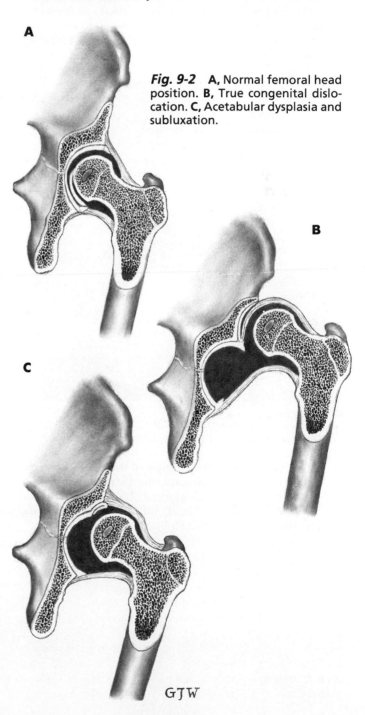

Fig. 9-2 **A,** Normal femoral head position. **B,** True congenital dislocation. **C,** Acetabular dysplasia and subluxation.

GJW

Correction of talipes equinovarus (clubfoot)

DESCRIPTION ■ A procedure involving posteromedial release of tight structures. These might include the Achilles tendon, subtalar joints, posterior tibialis, the calcaneonavicular and calcaneocuboid ligaments, and the calcaneocuboid joint.

INDICATIONS ■ Ineffective nonsurgical correction; adduction of the forefoot, inversion (varus) of the foot, and downward pointing of the foot and toes (equinus); shortened Achilles tendon; unilateral condition resulting in a smaller affected foot and calf; and/or contracted and thickened joint tissues in the ankle and foot, inhibiting function.

EQUIPMENT AND INSTRUMENTATION ■
Soft tissue instruments
Kirschner wires
Power equipment for pin insertion
Tourniquet

PROCEDURE ■

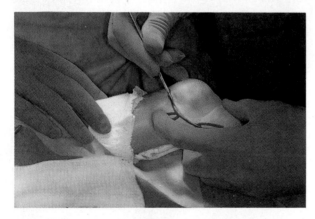

1 The patient is positioned prone on bilateral chest rolls with the head protected on a soft roll. Extremities are padded. A tourniquet is applied. Following a circumferential preparation of the extremity from the toes to the tourniquet, the extremity is draped and the incision site is marked. The incision is made from the base of the first metatarsal below the medial malleolus using a No. 15 blade.

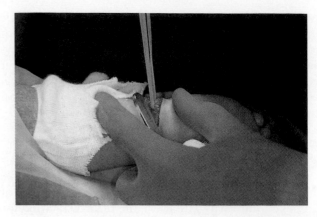

2 Following exposure of the Achilles tendon using scissors and forceps, a vessel loop is placed around the lesser saphenous vein and the sural nerve.

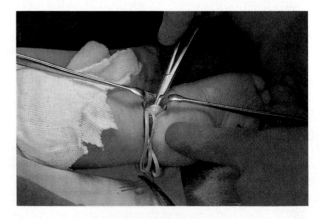

3 Ragnell retractors are placed for exposure. Iris scissors are used to expose the peroneus longus and brevis tendons.

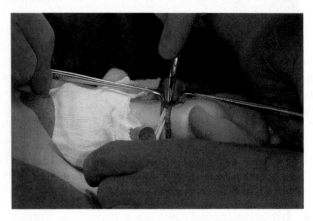

4 A curved mosquito hemostat is used to pass a vessel loop beneath the peroneus longus and brevis for retraction.

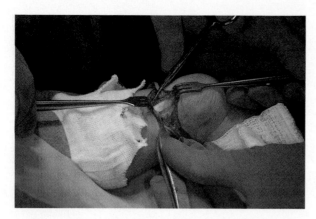

5 The distal Achilles tendon is exposed using Senn retractors.

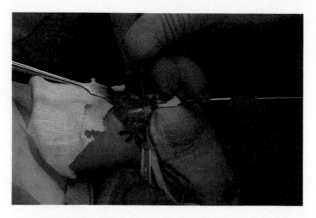

8 The Achilles tendon is exposed in the posterior midline, a Freer elevator is inserted between the tendon and the neurovascular bundle, and a Z lengthening cut is made using a No. 15 blade.

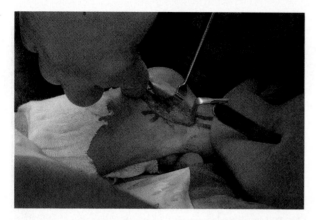

6 Iris scissors and forceps are used to dissect medially to the level of the deep fascia. The flexor tendon sheaths are opened, and the flexor digitorum longus and posterior tibial tendon are exposed. The blunt ends of the Senn retractors are used for exposure to protect the neurovascular bundle.

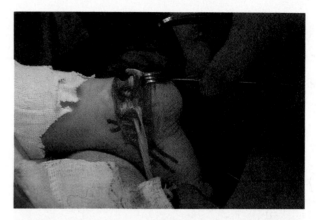

9 The Achilles tendon is cut in a Z-shaped manner (the proximal end of the distal stump is exposed). The posterior ankle joint and posterior subtalar joint are opened using Iris scissors (not pictured).

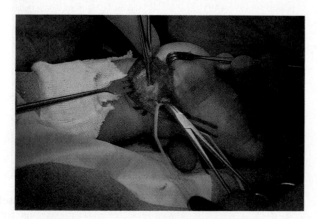

7 Following identification of the neurovascular bundle, a vessel loop is passed beneath for gentle retraction.

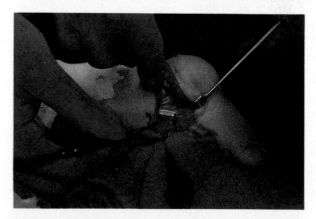

10 The posterior tibial tendon is resected using scissors. A Freer elevator is inserted over the dorsum of the talonavicular joint to retract the tibialis anterior and dorsalis pedis.

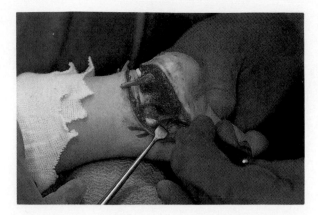

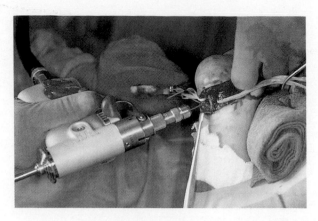

11   The talonavicular joint is exposed. The stump of the posterior tibial tendon is seen at the level of the blunt end of the Senn retractor, and the distal end of the Achilles tendon is seen at the posterior aspect of the wound.

14   A .054 Kirschner wire is inserted in the posterior aspect of the talus.

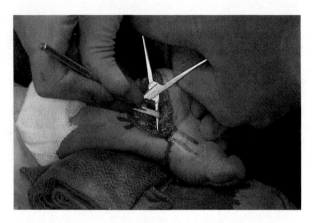

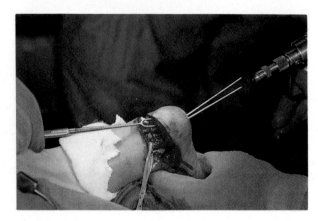

12   A Z lengthening of the flexor hallucis longus is completed by isolating the tendon with a mosquito hemostat and using a No. 64 Beaver blade. The Z lengthening is repaired using a 5-0 Prolene suture and Bishop forceps.

15   Two Kirschner wires are placed across the subtalar joint. The second pin is placed to control rotation. The skin edges are retracted with a skin hook to facilitate closure of the skin incision. Following placement of the wires, an absorbable suture is placed in the posterior tibial tendon.

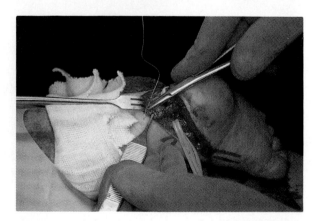

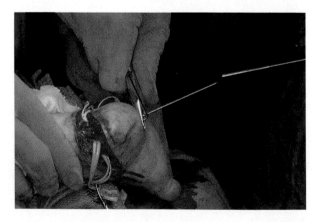

13   An absorbable suture is placed in the posterior tibial tendon.

16   The wires are bent with needle-nose pliers to prevent migration. The suction tip is used to complete a clean bend of the wire.

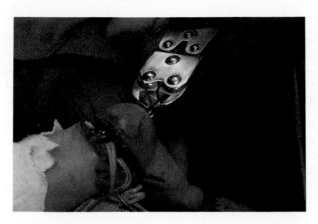

17 The pins are cut using a wire cutter, and the incision is irrigated.

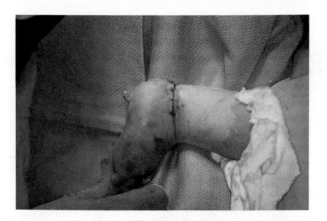

18 The lateral view shows a 90-degree angle to the leg.

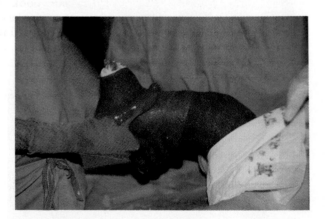

19 Following application of Steri-Strips, Xeroform, and an intermediate layer of dressing, a long leg cast is applied. Fiberglass layers are placed over a plaster cast to increase the cast's durability.

■ NURSING CARE AND TEACHING CONSIDERATIONS ■

Cast care is reinforced.
The cast is changed in 2 weeks; another long leg cast is applied.
The cast and Kirschner wire are removed at approximately 6 weeks postoperatively, and a third long leg cast is applied.
The cast is worn for approximately 4 months; an ankle-foot orthosis worn full or part time may be recommended for an additional 6 to 9 months.

Ilizarov method for treatment of bone defects

DESCRIPTION ■ A method of correction using closed reduction and establishing immobility with pins and ring configurations.

INDICATIONS ■ Bone defects caused by tumor, compound fractures, or debrided bone resulting from osteomyelitis; need for limb lengthening; nonunion fracture; open or closed fracture; or bony or soft tissue deformity.

EQUIPMENT AND INSTRUMENTATION ■
Soft tissue instruments
Ilizarov external fixator, consisting of a system of rings and semirings, connected with 1 mm pitch-threaded rods or telescoping rods (see Fig. 9-1)
Power equipment

PROCEDURE ■

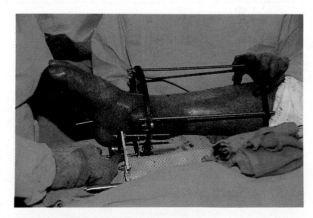

1 The patient is positioned appropriately for exposing the anatomic site. The leg is prepared and draped. Half-circle and full-circle rings are connected.

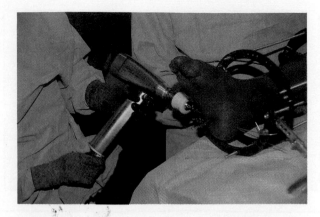

2 The fixator is applied using power equipment to insert 1.5 or 1.8 Kirschner wires. Fluoroscopy is used to determine the correct placement.

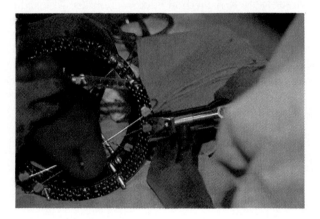

3 Rings, semirings, and rods are used to secure the placement of the fixation device.

■ **NURSING CARE AND TEACHING CONSIDERATIONS** ■

The patient's willingness to participate in rehabilitation and therapy must be ascertained before the procedure in order to enable a positive outcome. The success of the procedure depends on maintaining distraction protocol (usually every 6 hours). Weekly x-ray films are taken to determine whether distraction is occurring at the proper rate.

The bone is distracted at scheduled times of the day up to 1 mm per day beginning 5 to 7 days after the corticotomy.

Assess neurovascular status.

Reinforce pain therapy, including the medication regimen (severe pain may be experienced for the first 24 hours postoperatively).

Report unusual pain during distraction and any signs of neurologic impairment, such as numbness or tingling.

Teach pin site care, including cleansing with soap and water or hydrogen peroxide.

Correction of a congenital hip disorder

DESCRIPTION ■ May include repair of the capsule or an osteotomy with placement of internal fixation using pins or plates and screws.

INDICATIONS ■ Hip instability due to lack of acetabular depth or ligamentous laxity. Findings on examination include uneven knee height, uneven number of thigh skin folds, shortened thigh length, fullness of buttocks from posterior displacement of the femoral head, and asymmetric position of the greater trochanter.

EQUIPMENT AND INSTRUMENTATION ■
Small-bone instruments
Soft tissue instruments
Positioning supplies (sandbag)
Power equipment
Fixation devices

Open reduction
PROCEDURE ■

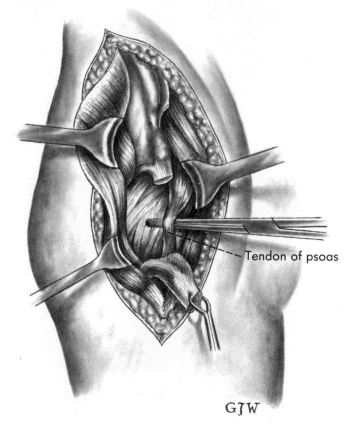

Tendon of psoas

GJW

1 The patient is placed in a semilateral position with the affected hip and buttock supported on a sandbag. The iliac crest is exposed, and the tendon of the psoas muscle is detached.

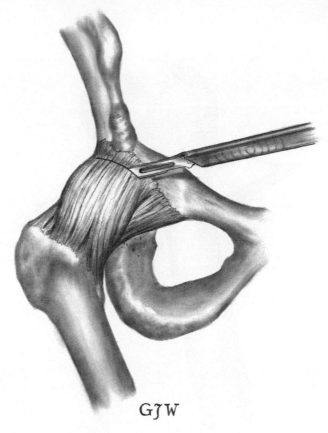

GJW

2 The capsule is dissected and opened using a knife blade. The joint is inspected for the causes of the dislocation.

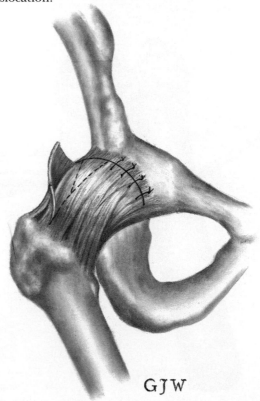

GJW

3 The femoral head is reduced and the capsule repaired by making an incision in the capsule to create a flap. Sutures are placed for repair. The specific repair is determined by the approach and the anatomic deformity of the hip.

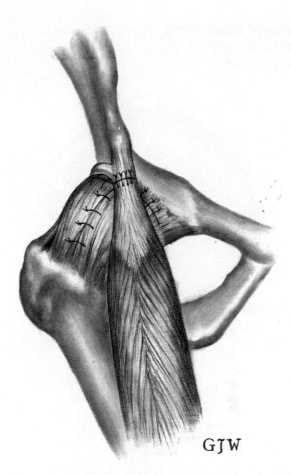

GJW

4 Following the repair, the rectus femoris is reattached, and the incision is closed.

<table>
<tr><td>■ NURSING CARE AND TEACHING CONSIDERATIONS ■</td></tr>
</table>

Teach cast care and limitations for a hip spica cast. The cast is applied and worn for a minimum of 10 to 12 weeks.

X-ray films are taken at 4 to 6 weeks postoperatively to determine the extent of correction. The portion of the cast below the knee may be removed to allow knee motion and some hip rotation.

After the cast has been worn for 10 to 12 weeks, an abduction brace may be worn for another 4 to 8 weeks, then only during sleep for 1 to 2 weeks.

Femoral osteotomy using a four-hole plate
PROCEDURE ■

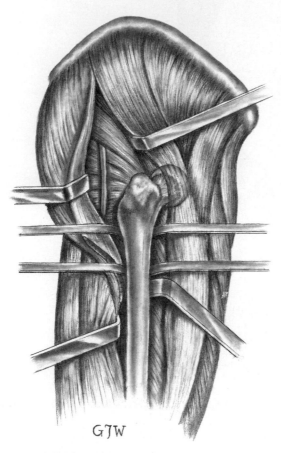

GJW

1 An incision is made to expose the femur. A self-retaining retractor is placed for exposure. Four spikes are inserted.

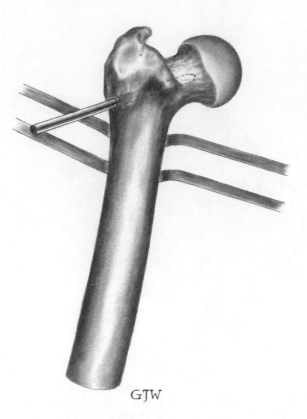

GJW

2 A Steinmann pin is inserted as a guide wire using power equipment.

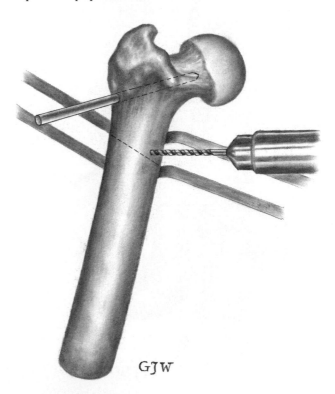

GJW

3 A drill hole is placed above the osteotomy line. The bone is divided using a blade. An osteotome is inserted between the cut surfaces.

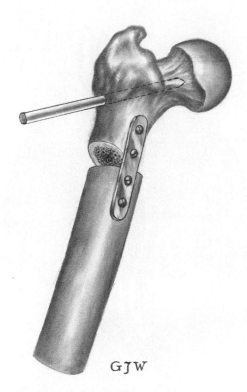

GJW

4 A four-hole plate is inserted. The Steinmann pin is removed. The tissue layers are closed.

Femoral osteotomy using a Coventry screw plate
PROCEDURE ■

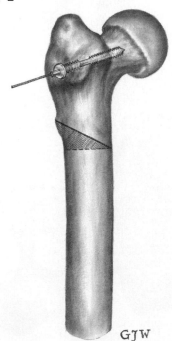

GJW

1 The patient is positioned supine. A Kirschner wire is inserted. The cortex is reamed, and a screw is inserted. A partial saw cut is made at the level of the lesser trochanter; a second saw cut is made to form a wedge. The osteotomy is complete, and the wedge is removed.

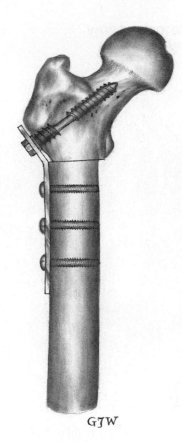

GJW

2 The plate and screw are inserted, and the incision is closed.

■ NURSING CARE AND TEACHING CONSIDERATIONS ■

Teach spica cast care.
Reinforce postoperative activities; immobilization may be required for 10 to 12 weeks.
Range of motion and full weight bearing with ambulation begins when the extent of healing is determined.

Innominate osteotomy
PROCEDURE ■

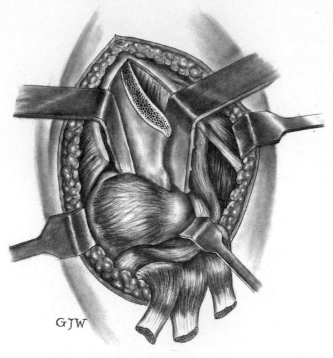

GJW

1 The patient is positioned semilaterally with a sandbag beneath the affected hip. The incision is made using a knife blade and/or cautery.

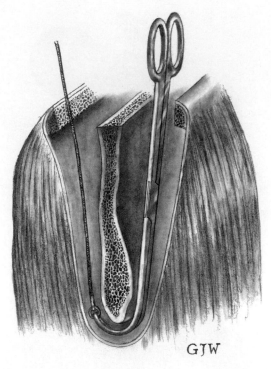

GJW

3 Curved (O'Shaughnessy) forceps are passed below the iliac crest, and a Gigli saw is received in the end of the forcep.

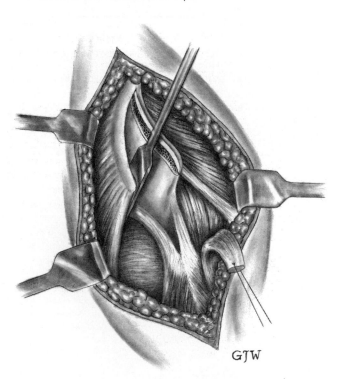

GJW

2 The wing of the ileum is exposed using a periosteal elevator. Large retractors are used to attain exposure. The tendon within the psoas muscle is incised. Joint stability is assessed. A long periosteal elevator is used to dissect the soft tissue.

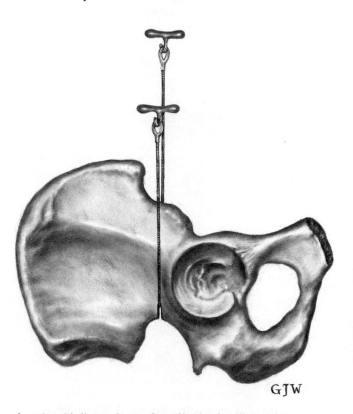

GJW

4 The Gigli saw is used to divide the iliac spine.

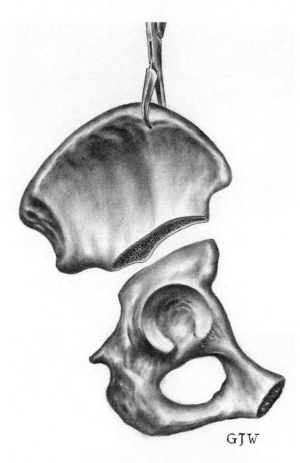

GJW

5 A holding clamp is used to displace fragments.

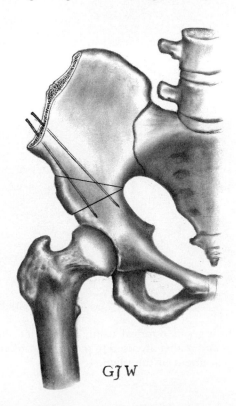

GJW

6 A bone graft is placed, and the position is stabilized using Kirschner wires or Steinmann pins. The capsule is repaired, and the incision is closed.

> ■ NURSING CARE AND TEACHING CONSIDERATIONS ■
>
> Teach cast care for the spica cast; the spica cast may remain in place for 10 to 12 weeks.
> Begin non-weight-bearing mobilization at 6 weeks, to continue for another 6 weeks.
> Range-of-motion exercises and full weight bearing may begin at 12 weeks.

Tibial osteotomy

DESCRIPTION ■ Realignment of the limb for transfer of weight bearing; a wedge of bone is removed above the tibial tuberosity.

INDICATIONS ■ Valgus deformity and collateral instability; pain; or degenerative changes of the knee.

EQUIPMENT AND INSTRUMENTATION ■
Soft tissue instruments
Large-bone instruments
Tourniquet
Power instruments
Instrumentation for placement of plate and screws

PROCEDURE ■

1 The patient is positioned supine, and the leg is prepared to include the upper thigh and foot. A U-drape is applied in a sterile manner. A stockinette is placed over the affected foot and rolled to cover the lower extremity. An extremity drape and iodophor-impregnated impervious sheet are applied.

2 Because of the minimal distance from the tourniquet site to the incision, sterile Webril padding is placed on the upper thigh before the tourniquet is placed. After the sterile tourniquet is placed, the extremity is elevated, and compression is applied using a sterile elastic bandage. The tourniquet pressure is elevated. The knee is slightly flexed during the procedure to relax the neurovascular structures.

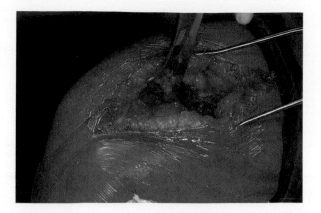

3 Following the incision with a No. 10 blade and deeper dissection using scissors and a cautery, Weitlaner retractors are placed for exposure.

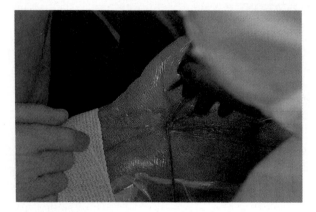

4 The guide pin is inserted using power equipment; depth is validated using fluoroscopy.

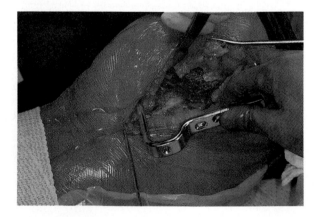

5 An angled plate is selected.

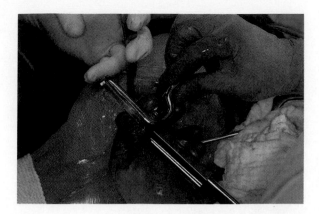

6 The chisel guide is placed on the seating chisel using a hexagonal screwdriver.

7 A positioning plate of the appropriate angle is used to evaluate the position.

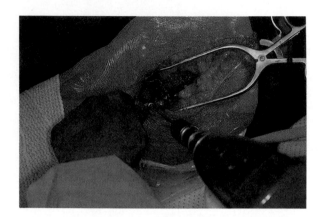

8 The Steinmann pin is inserted to mark the chisel cut site.

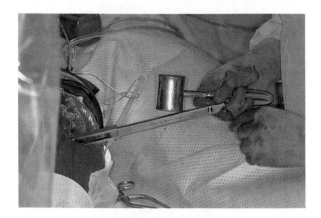

9 Following pin removal using pliers (not shown), a chisel and mallet are used to make the osteotomy cut for placement of the plate.

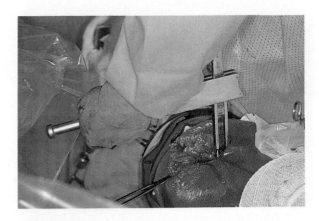

10   The chisel is removed using the extractor.

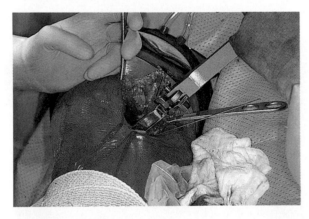

11   The plate is placed on the inserter-extractor, and the position is assessed.

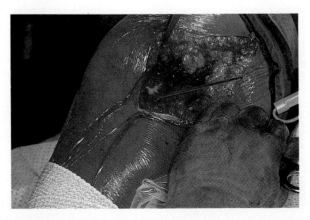

12   The pin is reinserted.

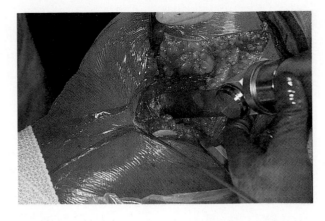

13   A wide blade is used to make an osteotomy cut.

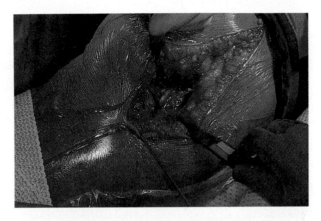

14   The osteotomy site is separated using manual pressure, and the wedge of bone is removed.

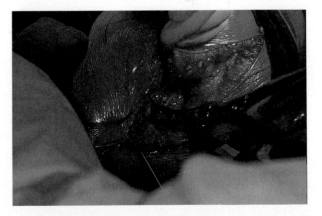

15   A Leksell rongeur is used to remove the bone.

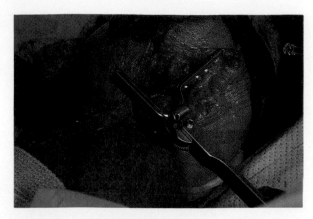

16 A wrench (not shown) is used to place the instrument extractor on the plate.

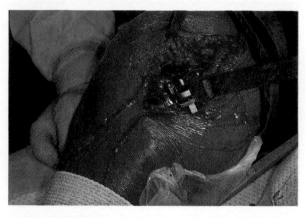

17 The 90-degree plate is positioned.

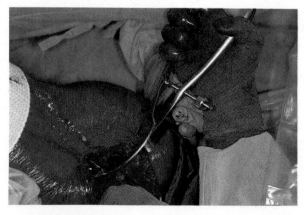

18 The plate is held in place using Lowman bone-holding forceps.

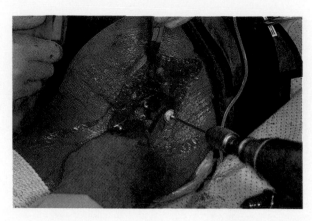

19 A drill guide is used with a 3.2 mm drill bit to prepare the screw holes.

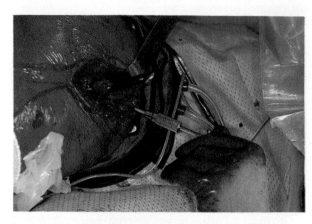

20 The depth gauge is used to measure screw length.

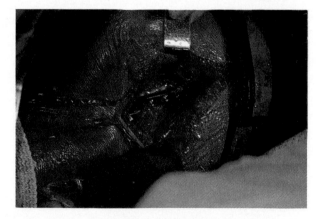

21 Screws are placed in each hole of the plate in the same manner.

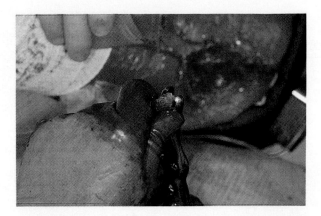

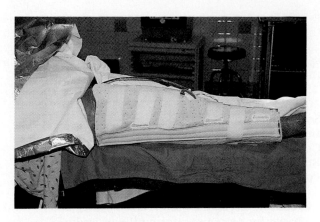

22 Bone previously removed from the surgical site is prepared by cutting it in small pieces. It is placed in the surgical site as bone graft.

26 The leg splint is placed.

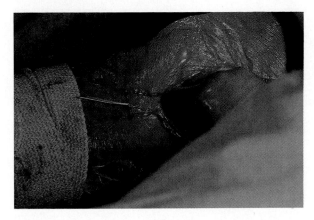

23 The drain is placed.

24 The incision site is closed with a heavy absorbable suture.

25 A dressing is applied.

■ NURSING CARE AND TEACHING CONSIDERATIONS ■

Observe for drainage.
Elevate the extremity for 24 to 48 hours to prevent swelling.
Encourage ambulation after 1 week.
- Full weight bearing and knee flexion begins after 1 week.
- Walking without the brace begins after 6 weeks.

SPINAL INSTRUMENTATION

Numerous techniques are used for instrumentation of the scoliotic spine. The anticipated outcome is to achieve a balanced, stable spine with minimal residual deformity. Instrumentation is placed for correction of the deformity and internal fixation. Approaches for spinal instrumentation include anterior and posterior approaches. The procedure selected varied with the specific need for correction and the instrumentation being used. When the anterior approach is used, a thoracic or general surgeon participates to attain exposure and manage postoperative care.

Treatment of vertebral deviation using the Cotrell Doubesset technique

DESCRIPTION ■ Internal fixation in the form of rods and hooks placed to maintain or improve alignment of the spine until a vertebral body fusion becomes solid. The system has the ability to distract and compress between segments with multiple hook placement.

INDICATIONS ■ Laterally deviated curve of the spine that does not demonstrate normal segmental mobility on lateral bending or distraction and increases in severity with nonoperative therapy; can also be performed for a thoracic spinal fracture.

EQUIPMENT AND INSTRUMENTATION ■
Soft tissue instruments
Instrumentation for laminectomy
Cotrell Doubesset Instrumentation
Bone-grafting instruments
Positioning supplies for the prone position

PROCEDURE ■ A bone graft is taken (see Chapter 7) and prepared for placement during the procedure.

1 The patient is positioned prone to expose the vertebrae for the procedure using a frame or chest rolls. Anatomic alignment is maintained during positioning. The airway is managed by turning the head to the side. The back is prepared from the cervical to the sacral vertebrae, and the area is draped. The bone graft site is also prepared.

2 A solution of epinephrine diluted to 1:500,000 is injected to reduce bleeding.

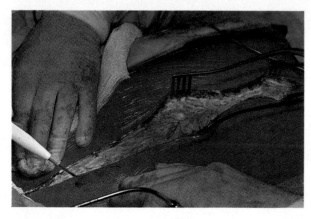

3 Following a midline incision using a No. 10 blade, exposure is maintained utilizing Weitlaner retractors to apply tension on soft tissues.

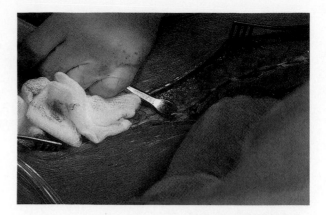

4 The spinous processes are exposed by stripping the tissue from the process using a cautery and Cobb elevator.

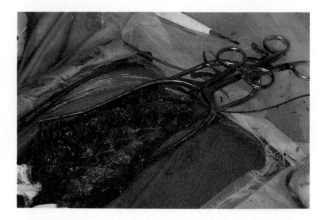

5 The spinous processes are removed using a rongeur, and the thoracic and lumbar areas are exposed.

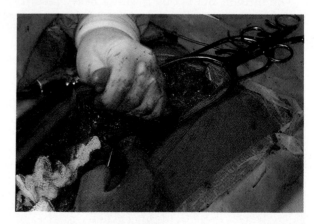

6 A notch is removed from an inferior facet in the thoracic region using an osteotome to prepare for hook site placement.

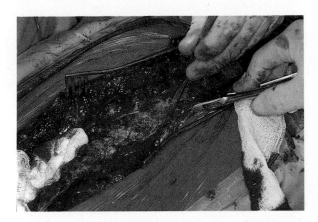

7   The rongeur is used to remove a small portion of the lamina for insertion of a hook into the sublaminar space.

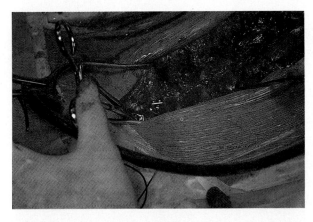

8   The hook is placed on the hook holder for placement into the sublaminar space.

9   The inferior hooks are placed.

10 A hook blocker is placed on a rod before the rod is contoured.

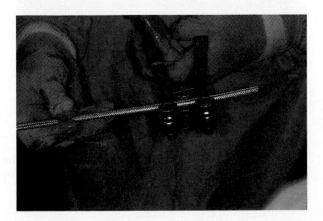

11 A rod bender is used to bend the rod.

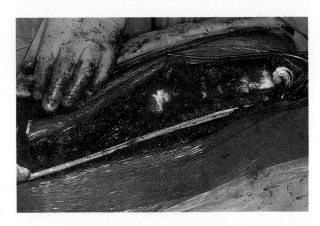

12 The rod is positioned to ensure adequate contouring and length before placement.

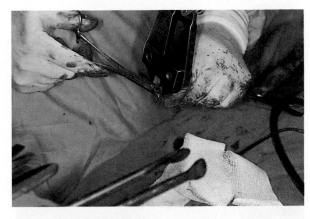

13 The bolt cutter is used to shorten the rod.

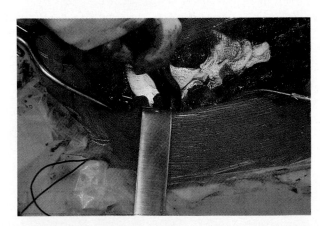

14 A small rongeur is used to decorticate bone and remove tissue.

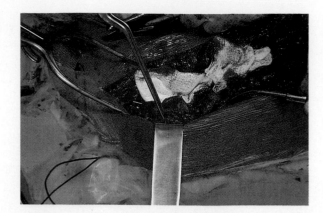

15 Bone graft, removed from the iliac crest, is placed along the decorticated surface outward to the transverse process in the lumbar and thoracic region using forceps.

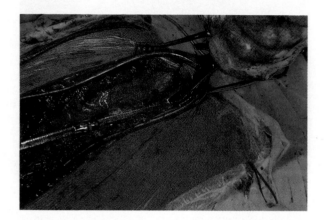

16 Following placement of the rod, a clamp and spreader are used to push the rod distally into the lower hooks.

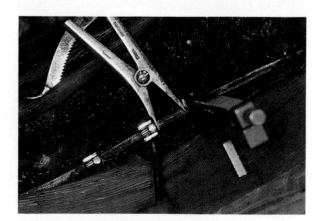

17 The hooks are secured using the hook blocker seated into the open hook. The clamp and spreader are used to spread the hook into its appropriate position.

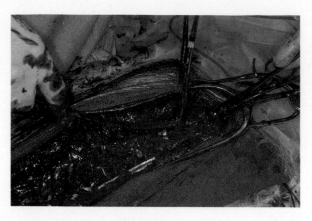

18 The rod is passed through the hooks.

19 A second rod is inserted and passed through the previously located hooks.

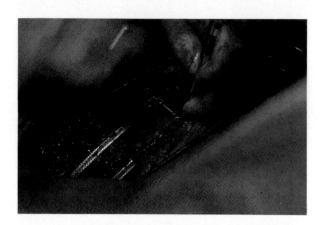

20 A cross-linking device is linked with both rods.

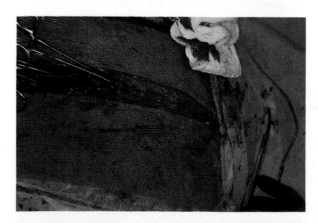

21 Towel clips are used to reapproximate the midline for closure.

22 The incision site is closed, and Steri-Strips are applied.

23 The dressing is applied, covering the midline incision site and the graft site.

> ■ **NURSING CARE AND TEACHING CONSIDERATIONS** ■
>
> Bed rest is required for approximately 12 hours postoperatively; sitting and bending are restricted.
>
> A fiberglass full-body brace may be applied at 24 hours postoperatively. The patient's activity level is gradually increased, and physical therapy begins. The cast may be worn for 4 to 6 months. Cast care is reinforced.
>
> Activities are gradually increased; complete resumption of activities is not expected for 1 year to allow bone growth.

Treatment of vertebral deviation using the Luque technique

DESCRIPTION ■ Internal fixation in the form of wires placed to maintain or improve alignment of the spine. Two L-shaped rods are inverted and placed so that they form a frame. Wires are passed beneath the laminae to secure each vertebra to the two metal rods.

INDICATIONS ■ Laterally deviated curve of the spine that does not demonstrate normal segmental mobility on lateral bending; or distraction increasing in severity with nonoperative therapy.

EQUIPMENT AND INSTRUMENTATION ■
Soft tissue instruments
Luque instrumentation
Positioning supplies for the prone position

PROCEDURE ■

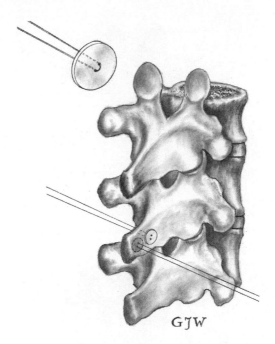

1 The patient is positioned prone. Following exposure of the vertebrae, wires are passed through a Drummond button and through the base of the spinous process.

2 Rods are initially bent at the angle anticipated for the desired degree of reduction.

3 The spinous processes are excised with a rongeur.

4 Facet joints are resected using a rongeur.

5   Sublaminar wires are passed.

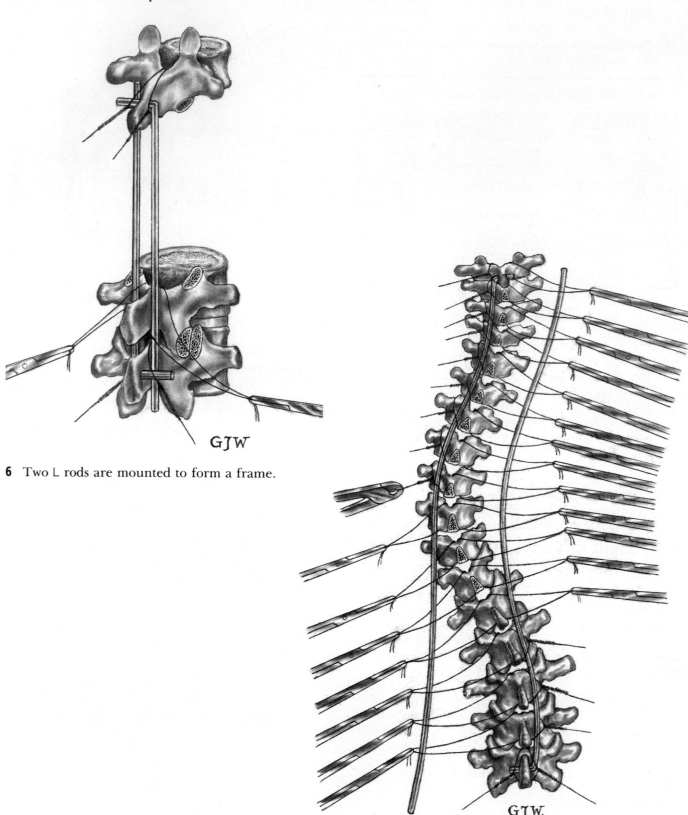

6   Two L rods are mounted to form a frame.

7   Wires are tightened on the rod for correction of the curvature.

8 The frame is secured, bleeding is maintained, and the incision site is closed.

■ **NURSING CARE AND TEACHING CONSIDERATIONS** ■

Mobilization begins usually within 36 hours. A postoperative corset or splint may be deemed necessary depending on the fixation.
Normal activities may be resumed by 6 months

Dwyer and Zielke procedures

DESCRIPTION ■ Procedures performed through an anterolateral approach on the convex side of the curve. Dwyer and Zielke procedures may be chosen when the posterior approach is insufficient. Dwyer instrumentation was developed in 1964 for correction of lordosis and fixation through the anterior approach. Zielke modified Dwyer's principles by changing the type of rods, allowing for correction of kyphotic areas of the spine. This cannot be accomplished using the Dwyer system.

INDICATIONS ■ Selected spinal deformities, including the following: a lumbar curves in patients with deficient posterior elements such as myelomeningocele; thoracolumbar curves with extreme lordosis; and rigid thoracocolumbar paralytic curves for which a combined anteroposterior fusion in two stages is required.

INSTRUMENTATION ■
Dwyer instrumentation uses large metal staples of several sizes that are attached to each vertebral body with a large screw. The screws have large heads with holes for passage of a cable that is tightened at each level and fixed by crimping the screw heads.
The **Zielke system** is a modification of the Dwyer instrumentation. Implants are made of stainless steel with slotted screw heads. Screws are implanted into the vertebral bodies through convex circular washers or angled plates. A solid flexion rod replaces the cable used in the Dwyer instrumentation.

Dwyer
PROCEDURE ■

1 The patient is placed in the lateral decubitus position. Disks are excised.
2 The staple is inserted around the body of the vertebra.
3 A screw is inserted through the staple and into the vertebral body. A screwdriver and tensioner are used to remove slack and to tighten the cable between the screws.
4 Correction is attained.

Zielke
PROCEDURE ■

1 Following exposure, Zielke screws and washers are inserted through the appropriate vertebral bodies. A threaded rod is applied through screw heads.
2 The spine is derotated, and lordosis is applied for correction.

■ **NURSING CARE AND TEACHING CONSIDERATIONS** ■

Assess for postoperative complications related to the anterior surgical approach, including pneumothorax, hemothorax, aspiration pneumonia, and paralytic ileus.
Include consideration of the proximity to the spinal cord and possible related complications in the postoperative assessment.

BIBLIOGRAPHY

Association of Operating Room Nurses, Inc.: *AORN standards and recommended practices for perioperative nursing—1992*, Denver, 1992, AORN.
Canale TS, Beaty JH: *Operative pediatric orthopaedics*, St Louis, 1991, Mosby.
Chapman MW: *Operative orthopedics*, vols 1 and 2, Philadelphia, 1988, JB Lippincott.
Crenshaw AH: *Campbell's operative orthopaedics*, vols 1 through 5, ed 8, St Louis, 1992, Mosby.
Evarts CM: *Surgery of the musculoskeletal system*, ed 2, New York, 1990, Churchill Livingstone.
Gaehle K and others: Adult lumbar scoliosis: treatment with combined anterior-posterior spinal fusion, *AORN J* 54:546, Sept 1991.
Laurin C, Riley LH, Roy-Camille R: *Atlas of orthopaedic surgery*, vols 1 and 3, St Louis, 1992, Mosby.
Meeker M, Rothrock J: *Alexander's care of the patient in surgery*, ed 9, St Louis, 1991, Mosby.
Mercier LR: *Practical orthopedics*, St Louis, 1991, Mosby.
Preksto D: The Kaneda device: a new anterior spine stabilization system, *AORN J* 55:734, March 1992.
Renshaw TS: The role of Harrington instrumentation and posterior spine fusion in the management of adolescent idiopathic scoliosis, *Orthop Clin North Am* 19:257, April 1988.
Rosman M, Brown K: Preoperative Ilizarov frame construction for correction of ankle and foot deformities, *Pediatr Orthop* 11:238, 1991.
Rothrock J: *Perioperative nursing care planning*, St Louis, 1990, Mosby.
Silverman BJ, Greenburg PE: Idiopathic scoliosis posterior spine fusion with Harrington rod and sublaminar wiring, *Orthop Clin North Am* 19:269, April 1988.

Index

A

Absorbable pin, 58
Abuse, victims of, 30
Ace-Fischer fixator, 154
Acetabulum, 20
Acid phosphatase, 34
Acquired musculoskeletal disorders, 73-143
Acromioclavicular joint, 17, 18
Acromion process of scapula, 17, 18
Adaptic gauze, 67
Adson cerebellum retractors, 52
Adson periosteal elevator, 49
Adson rongeur, 50
Adults, older
  nursing care for, 30
  physical changes in, 30
Agee wrist jack, 154
Airflow and infection control, 42
Alkaline phosphatase, 34
Allografts, 140-141
Alm retractor, 53
Amphiarthroses, 11, 12
Amphiarthrotic joints, 11, 12
Amputation saw, 57
Anatomic neck of humerus, 18
Andry, Nicholas, 4
Anesthesia team, role of, 6
Anesthesiologist, 6
Anesthetics, 36-37
Anesthetist, registered nurse, certified, 6
Ankle arthroscopy, 89-91
Annulus fibrosus, 14
Anterior cervical discectomy and fusion, 104-108
Anterior cruciate ligament reconstruction, arthroscopic, with patellar tendon substitution, 78-83
Anteroposterior views, 62
Antibiotics and infection control, 43
Antinuclear antibody test, 34
AO external fixation device, 147
AO fixation device, 146
AO frame pin fixator system, 154
AO interlocked fixation device, 146
AO Universal fixation device, 146
Appendicular skeleton, 11, 12

Appliances, external fixation with, 154-160
Aprons, leaded, for radiography, 63
Arches of foot, 23, 25
Arthritis, rheumatoid, arthroplasty for, 111
Arthrodial joint, 14
Arthrography, 32-33
Arthroplasty, 111-134
  hip, 122-129
  Keller resection, 137-138
  metacarpophalangeal joint implant, 112-113
  shoulder joint, 118-122
  total elbow joint, 113-118
Arthroscopic anterior cruciate ligament reconstruction with patellar tendon substitution, 78-83
Arthroscopic knee procedures, position for, 39
Arthroscopy (arthroscopic procedures), 74-91
  ankle, 89-91
  diagnostic, 75
  equipment and instrumentation specific for, 75
  knee, diagnostic or operative, 75-78
  operative, 75
  shoulder, 83-86
Articular cartilage, 12, 13
Articular disk, 12
Articular process, 15, 16
Articulation
  radioulnar, 12
  tibiofibular, 12
Aspartate aminotransferase, serum, 34
Aspiration
  bone marrow, 33
  joint, 33
Assessment of patient by perioperative nurse, 31-34
Assistive support personnel, role of, 7
Association of Operating Room Nurses, quality improvement standards for perioperative nursing, 43
Atlas vertebra, 16
Aufranc cobra retractor, 52
Austin Moore prosthetic replacement for femoral head, 173
Autogenous bone grafts, 140
Awls, bone, 53
Axial skeleton, 11, 12
Axillary block, 37
Axis vertebra, 16

B

Baby Inge bone spreader, 52
Bacterial osteomyelitis, 45
Ball-and-socket joint, 13, 14
Bankart procedure, 97-99
Barton's fracture, 150
Beckman-Adson retractor, 53
Bending clamp, 53
Bending pliers, 53
Bending press, 53
Bennett retractor, 52
Bennett's fracture, 150
Berndt hip ruler, 55
Biceps muscle, 18
Bicondylar tibial plateau fracture, 186
Bier block, 37
Bilateral process, 15
Biopsy, bone marrow, 33
Blades and burs, 56
Block, anesthetic, 37
Blood specimens, testing of, 33
Blood supply of bone, 9, 10
Blood tests, 33
Blount double-pronged retractor, 52
Blount nylon mallet, 54
Blount single-pronged retractor, 52
Bodysuits, 64
Bone(s); *see also* specific bone
    blood vessels in, 9, 10
    classification of, by shape, 9, 11
    defects of, Ilizarov method for treatment of, 197-198
    development and healing of, 26-27
    of foot, 23-24
    growth of, 26-27
    healing of, 27
    structure of, 9, 10
    types of, 9
Bone awls, 53
Bone banks, 140-141
Bone clamps, 52
Bone curettes, 50
Bone graft, 141-142
    cancellous, 141
    cortical, 142
    materials for, properties of, 140
    and stimulation, 140-142
Bone hook, 51
Bone marrow aspiration or biopsy, 33
Bone rasps, 51
Bone scintigraphy, 33
Bone screw ruler gauge, 55
Bone screws, 162-163
Bone spreader, 52
Bone stimulation, 142
Bone tamps, 54
Bone-cutting forceps, 51
Bone-holding instruments, 51-52
Braces, 67
Bristow-Helfet shoulder repair, modified, 101
Brooker-Wells fixation device, 146
Brun bone curette, 50
Bunions, surgical procedures for, 135
Burs, blades and, 56
Bursae, 12, 14
    of knee, 23
Bursectomy of olecranon, 95-96

C

Calcaneus bone, 25
Calcium, serum, 34
Caliper, 55
Callus and bone healing, 27
Cancellous bone, 9
Cancellous bone graft, 141
Cancellous screws, 57, 58, 146, 163
Cannulated wire cutter, 54
Capitate bone, 19
Capitellum of humerus, 18
Capsulorrhaphy for anterior shoulder repair, 97-99
Cardiac muscle, 25
Carpal bones, 19
Carpal tunnel release, 94-95
    endoscopic, 86-88
Carpus, 19
Cartilage(s)
    articular, 12, 13
    costal, 16, 17
Cast(s)
    application of, 153, 154
    materials for, 65-66
    removal of, 66
Cast saw, 66
Cavity, glenoid, 17
Cellular proliferation and bone healing, 27
Cement, PMMA, reactions to, 66
Cement gun to inject PMMA, 67
Certified registered nurse anesthetist, 6
Certified surgical technologist, role of, 6
Cervical curvature, 15
Cervical discectomy and fusion, anterior, 104-108
Cervical vertebrae, 14, 15, 16
Chandler elevator, 49
Charnley, John, 4
Chest, 16-17
Chevron distal metatarsal osteotomy, 135-136
Children, nursing care for, 29-30
Chisels, 49
Chuck key, 55
    hand drills and, 56
Chucks, 55
Circlage, 161
Circumferential wire fixation, 161
Clamp(s)
    bending, 53
    bone, 52
Clamp fixators, external fixation with, 154
Clavicle, 17, 18
Cleansing, skin, and infection control, 42
Cleavage fracture, fixation of 186-187
Clinical practice, perioperative nursing, standards of, 29
Closed fractures, 151
Closed reduction of fracture, 152-153
Clubfoot; *see* Talipes equinovarus
Cobb spinal elevator, 49
Cobb spinal gouges, 49
Coccygeal vertebrae, 14, 16
Coccyx, 16
Collagen and bone healing, 27
Collarbone, 17-18
Collateral ligaments of knee, 23
Colles' fracture, 150
Comminuted fracture, 151, 152

Comminuted subtrochanteric fracture, 175
Communication
  with patients, 30-31
  postoperative, 69
Compact bone, 9, 10
Compartment pressure monitor, 147
Compartment syndrome, 45
Compressed air equipment, 55-56
Compression fracture, 151, 152
Compression plate fixation of forearm fracture, 164-167
Compression side plate and screw, insertion of, 178-182
Compression slot, fixation plate with, 146
Computed tomography, 33
Condyles
  of femur, 21
  of tibia, 21
Condyloid joint, 13, 14
Congenital anomalies, 191-213
  common, procedures for, 193-207
  nursing care for, 191-193
  nursing diagnoses related to, 191-192
  spinal instrumentation for, 207-213
Congenital hip disorders, correction of, 193, 198-199
Coracoid process of scapula, 17-18
Coronoid fossa, 18
Correction, hammertoe, 139-140
Cortical bone, 9
Cortical bone graft, 142
Cortical bone screws, 162
Cortical screws, 57, 58, 146
Costal cartilages, 16, 17
Cotrell Doubesset technique for treatment of vertebral deviation, 207-213
Cotton's fracture, 150
Coventry screw plate, femoral osteotomy using, 201
Coxae, 20
Craig biopsy needle, 33
C-reactive protein, 34
Creatinine phosphokinase, 34
Cross-slot screw, 58
Cruciate ligament of knee, 23
  anterior, arthroscopic reconstruction of, with patellar tendon substitution, 78-83
CT; see Computed tomography
Cuboid bone, 25
Cuneiform bones, 23, 25
Curettes, 50
Curves of spinal column, 15
Cushing elevator, 49
Cutters, 54
Cutting instruments, 48-51

D

DCP fixation plate, 146
Deep venous thrombosis, 44-45
Dens of axis vertebra, 16
Depressed plateau fracture, fixation of, 187-188
Depressed tibial plateau fracture, 186
Depth gauges, 55
Deviation, vertebral, treatment of
  using Cotrell Doubesset technique, 207-211
  using Luque technique, 211-213
Diagnoses, nursing, 34
  related to acquired musculoskeletal disorders, 73-74
  related to congenital anomalies, 191-192
  related to traumatic musculoskeletal injury, 148-149

Diagnostic arthroscopy, 75
Diagnostic knee arthroscopy, 75-78
Diagnostic procedures
  invasive, 32-33
  noninvasive, 33-34
  required before orthopaedic procedures, 32-34
Diamond pin cutter, 54
Diarthroses, 12, 13, 14
Diarthrotic joints, 12, 13
  types of, 14
Discectomy, anterior cervical, and fusion, 104-108
Disk(s)
  articular, 12
  intervertebral, 14, 15
  removal of, lumbar laminectomy for, 108-111
Documentation of care, 41
  for congenital anomalies, 192
  for traumatic musculoskeletal injury, 149
Dorsal recumbent position, 39
Double-contrast arthrography, 32-33
Double-ended Putti bone rasp, 51
Drainage systems, wound, 67
Draping and infection control, 42-43
Dressings, 67, 68
  hot ice incorporated in, 67, 68
Drills, 56
Dwyer instrumentation, 213
Dwyer procedure, 213

E

Elbow, external fixation of, 157-161
Elbow joint arthroplasty, total, 113-118
Electromyography, 33
Elevators, 49
Ellipsoidal joint, 13, 14
Embolism
  fat, 44
  pulmonary, 45
EMG; see Electromyography
Endarthrodial joint, 13, 14
Endoprosthesis for hemiarthroplasty, 176
Endoscopic carpal tunnel release, 86-88
Endosteum, 9
Epicondyles of femur, 18, 21
Epidural anesthesia, 36-37
Epiphyseal growth plate, function of, 26-27
Epiphyses of bone, 9
Eponyms for fractures, 150-151
Equipment
  arthroscopic, 75
  compressed air, 55-56
  documentation of use of, 41
  radiographic, 61-63
  required for orthopaedic procedures, 36
  and supplies, 61-69
  types of, 61-69
Erythrocyte sedimentation rate, 34
Evaluation, nursing, 43-45
Exsanguination, 63
External fixation
  with appliances, 154-161
  complications of, 154
  of elbow, 157-161
  of forearm, 155-157
External fixation devices, 147
External fixator, Ilizarov, 193

Extremity
lower, 20-25
muscles of, 26
upper, 18-19
muscles of, 25

F

False pelvis, 20
False ribs, 17
Fat embolism syndrome, 44
Femoral neck fractures, 172, 174
multiple pin fixation of, 177-178
Femoral osteotomy
using Coventry screw plate, 201
using four-hole plate, 200-201
Femoral shaft fractures, 176
Femur, 20-21
fracture of, management of, 172-176
head of, blood supply to, 173
intramedullary rodding of, 182-185
Ferris-Smith modified Kerrison rongeur, 50
Fibrin network and bone healing, 27
Fibroblasts and bone healing, 27
Fibula, 21, 22-23
Finger, trigger, release of, 92-93
First assistant, registered nurse, role of, 6, 36
Fixation
of cleavage fracture, 186-187
compression plate, of forearm fracture, 164-167
of depressed plateau fracture, 187-188
external; *see* External fixation
internal; *see* Internal fixation
pin, multiple, of femoral neck fracture, 177-178
screws for, 146
wire, circumferential, 161
Fixation devices
application of, 153-176
external, 147
intramedullary, 146
Fixation plates, 146
Fixator(s)
external, Ilizarov, 193
pin and ring, external fixation with, 154
Flat bones, 11
Flexor hallucis longus tendon, 25
Floating ribs, 17
Fluids, abnormal, testing of, 33
Fluoroscopy equipment, 62
Foot
arches of, 23, 25
bones of, 23-24
disorders of, procedures to correct, 135-140
Foramen (foramina)
intervertebral, 14, 15
nutrient, 9
obturator, 20
pelvic, 16
vertebral, 15
Forceps, bone-cutting, 51
Forearm
bones of, 18-19
external fixation of, 155-157
fracture of, compression plate fixation of, 164-167
Fossa
coronoid, 18
iliac, 20

Fossa—cont'd
intercondylar, 21
olecranon, 18
radial, 18
Four-hole plate, femoral osteotomy using, 200-201
Fovea capitis, 21
Fracture(s)
cleavage, fixation of 186-187
closed reduction of, 152-153
femoral, management of, 172-176
femoral neck, 172, 174
multiple pin fixation of, 177-178
femoral shaft, 176
forearm, compression plate fixation of, 164-167
intertrochanteric, compression side plate and screw insertion
for, 178-182
management of, goals of, 149
metacarpal, open reduction and internal fixation of, 167-169
patellar, repair of, 169-172
plateau, depressed, fixation of, 187-188
proper names (eponyms) for, 150-151
prosthetic shoulder replacement for, 122
tibial plateau, management of, 186
treatment of, 151-188
types of, 151, 152
Fracture reduction, 62
Fracture table, 65, 147
Freer elevator-dissector, 49
Fusion, anterior cervical diskectomy and, 104-108
Fusion site stimulator, insertion of, 142

G

Galeazzi's fracture, 150
Galen, 3
Garden's classification of femoral neck fractures, 172, 174
Gauges, depth, 55
Gigli saw, 57
Ginglymoid joint, 13, 14
Glenoid cavity, 17
Glenoid labrum, 21
Glenoid osteotomy, 103
Glenoplasty, 103
Gliding joint, 13, 14
Gloves, 64
Gluteal lines, 20
Gluteal muscles, 20
Goniometers, 55
Gouges, 49
Graft, bone, 140-142
cancellous, 141
cortical, 142
materials for, properties of, 140
Granulation tissue and bone healing, 27
Greater pelvis, 20
Greater trochanter, 21
Greater tubercle, 18
Grosse-Kampf interlocked fixation device, 146
Growth plate, epiphyseal, function of, 26-27

H

Hallux valgus, surgical procedures for, 135
Hamate bone, 19
Hammertoe correction, 139-140
Hand drill and chuck key, 56
Hand saws, 57
Healing, bone, 27

Heel bone, 23, 25
Hematoma and bone healing, 27
Hemiarthroplasty, 176-177
Hemilaminectomy, 104
Herbert bone screw, 162, 163
Hexagonal-slot screw, 58
Hibbs chisel, 49
Hibbs gouges, 49
Hibbs osteotome, 49
Hibbs retractor, 52
Hinge joint, 13, 14
Hip, congenital disorder of, correction of, 193, 198-199
Hip arthroplasty, 122-129
Hip bones, 20
Hip joint, 21
Hip replacement, total, 122-129
History of orthopaedic surgery, 3-4
Hoffmann fixator, 154
Hohmann retractor, 52
Hoods, 64
Hook, bone, 51
Hot ice incorporated in dressing, 67, 68
Humerus, 18
Hunchback; *see* Kyphosis

I
Iliac crest, 20
   bone graft of, 141
Iliac fossa, 20
Iliac spines, 20
Iliac tuberosity, 20
Iliofemoral ligament, 21
Ilium, 20
Ilizarov external fixator, 193
Ilizarov frame, 154
Ilizarov method for treatment of bone defects, 197-198
Imaging, magnetic resonance, 33
Immobilizers, 68
Implant(s)
   metacarpophalangeal joint, arthroplasty for, 112-113
   orthopaedic, 57-58
Implantable devices, assessment for presence of, 32
Implementation in nursing process, 38-43
Infections, wound, 45
   control of, 41-43
Inferior articular process, 15, 16
Inflammation and bone healing, 27
Infraglenoid tubercle, 17
Infraspinous muscle, 18
Injury, musculoskeletal, traumatic, 145-189; *see also* Traumatic
   musculoskeletal injury
Innominate bone, 20
Innominate osteotomy, 202-203
Instruments (instrumentation), 47-59
   arthroscopic, 75
   basic, 48
   bone-holding, 51-52
   care and handling of, 47-48
   cleaning of, 47
   cutting, 48-51
   microsurgery, 66
   misuse of, 47
   nonspecific, 53-58
   power-driven, 55-56
   retracting, 52, 53
   soft tissue, basic, 48

Instruments (instrumentation)—cont'd
   spinal, for congenital anomalies, 207-213
   to treat traumatic musculoskeletal injury, 145-147
Intercondylar fossa, 21
Interlocked fixation devices, 146
Internal fixation, 161-163
   circumferential wire fixation for, 161
   using Kirschner wires, 161, 162
   nail-and-plate combinations for, 163-164
   nails for, 163, 164
   open reduction and, of metacarpal fractures, 167-169
   plates for, 163
   rods for, 163, 164
   screws for, 162-163
   Steinmann pins for, 161
Interscalene block, 37
Intertrochanteric crest, 21
Intertrochanteric fractures, 172, 175
   compression side plate and screw insertion for, 178-182
Intertrochanteric line, 21
Intertubercular groove, 18
Intervertebral disks, 14, 15
Intervertebral foramina, 14, 15
Intramedullary fixation devices, 146
Intramedullary rodding of femur, 182-185
Intraoperative planning, 37-38
Intraoperative policies and procedures, 37-38
Intravenous regional anesthesia, 37
Invasive diagnostic procedures, 32-33
Irregular bones, 11
Ischium, 20

J
Joint(s), 11-14
   acromioclavicular, 17, 18
   classification of, 11-12
   elbow; *see* Elbow joint
   hip, 21
   knee, 22
   metacarpophalangeal; *see* Metacarpophalangeal joint
   movements at, 14
   sacroiliac, 20
   shoulder; *see* Shoulder joint
   types of, 11-12, 14
Joint aspiration, 33
Joint capsule, 12, 13
Joint Commission on Accreditation of Healthcare Organizations,
   43

K
Keine bone tamp, 54
Keller resection arthroplasty, 137-138
Kern bone-holding forceps, 51
Key periosteal elevator, 49
Kirschner wires, 58
   internal fixation using, 161, 162
Knee arthroplasty, 129-134
Knee arthroscopy, diagnostic or operative, 75-78
Knee joint, 22
   ligaments of, 23
Knee procedures, arthroscopic, position for, 39
Knee replacement, total, 129-134
Knee-chest position, modifications of, 41
Kneecap, 20, 21, 23
Kocher, Theodor, 4

Küntscher fixation device, 146
Kyphosis, 15

L

Laboratory tests, 32, 33
Lactic dehydrogenase, 34
Lag screws, 146
Lambotte-type osteotomes, 49
Laminar airflow, 42
Laminectomy, 104
   lumbar, for disk removal, 108-111
Lane bone-holding forceps, 51
Langenbeck periosteal elevator, 49
Lasers, 66
Lateral decubitus position, 39-40
Lateral views, 62
LE cell prep, 34
Leaded aprons or shields for radiography, 63
Leg holder, 65
Leksell rongeur, 50
Lesser pelvis, 20
Lesser trochanter, 21
Lesser tubercle, 18
Lewin bone-holding clamp, 52
Ligament(s), 9, 14
   cruciate, anterior, arthroscopic reconstruction of, with patellar
      tendon substitution, 78-83
   iliofemoral, 21
   of knee, 23
   patellar, 23
Ligamenta flava, 14-15
Ligamentum teres, 21
Linea aspera femoris, 21
Liston bone-cutting forceps, 51
Long bones, 9, 11
Long-bone stimulator, insertion of, 142
Longitudinal arches of foot, 23, 25
Lordosis, 15
Lower extremity, 20-25
   muscles of, 26
Lowman bone clamp, 52
Lumbar curvature, 15
Lumbar laminectomy for disk removal, 108-111
Lumbar vertebrae, 14, 15, 16
Lunate bone, 19
Luque technique for treatment of vertebral deviation, 211-213

M

Magnetic resonance imaging, 33
Magnuson-Stack shoulder repair, 102
Malgaigne's fracture, 150
Malleolus, lateral and medial, 22-23
Mallets, 54
Manual saws, 57
Manubrium, 17
Marrow, bone
   aspiration or biopsy of, 33
   distribution of, 10
   types of, 9
Masks with shields, 64
Measuring devices, 55
Medical status, assessment of, 31
Medullary cavity, 10
Membrane, synovial, 13
Meniscus, 12
   of knee joint, 23

Metacarpal bones, 19
Metacarpal fractures, open reduction and internal fixation of,
   167-169
Metacarpophalangeal joint implant arthroplasty, 112-113
Metatarsal bones, 23, 25
Metatarsal osteotomy, Chevron distal, 135-136
Meyerding laminectomy retractor, 53
Microscopes, 66
Microsurgery instruments, 66
Mixed tibial plateau fracture, 186
Modified Bristow-Helfet shoulder repair, 101
Monitor, pressure, compartment, 147
Monteggia's fracture, 150
Monticelli Spinelli fixator, 154
MRI; *see* Magnetic resonance imaging
Multiple pin fixation of femoral neck fracture, 177-178
Muscles, 24, 25, 26; *see also* specific muscle
   of arm, 25
   fibers of, 25-26
   of lower extremity, 26
   rotator cuff, 18
   structure of, 25-26
   of trunk, 24
   types of, 25
Musculoskeletal disorders, acquired, 73-143
Musculoskeletal injury, traumatic, 145-189; *see also* Traumatic
      musculoskeletal injury
Musculoskeletal structures, 9-27
Myelogram, 33

N

Nail-and-plate combinations for internal fixation, 163-164
Nails, 57, 58
   for internal fixation, 163, 164
Navicular bone, 23, 25
Needle, Craig biopsy, 33
Needle biopsy of bone marrow, 33
Needle-nose pliers and cutter, 54
Neer fracture, 151
Neural arch of vertebra, 15
Neuroma resection, 91-92
Neutralization fixation plate, 146
Noninvasive bone stimulation, 142
Noninvasive diagnostic procedures, 33-34
Non-self-tapping screw, 162
North American Nursing Diagnosis Association, 34
Nucleus pulposus, 14
Nurse
   orthopaedic, perioperative, role of, 5-6
   registered; *see* Registered nurse
Nursing
   perioperative
      AORN quality improvement standards for, 43
      clinical practice of, standards of, 29
   surgical, orthopaedic, foundations of, 1-69
Nursing activities and infection control, 42
Nursing assessment, 31-34
Nursing care
   for acquired musculoskeletal disorders, 73-74
   for congenital anomalies, 191-193
   perioperative, 29-46
   for special populations, 29-30
   for traumatic musculoskeletal injury, 145
Nursing diagnoses, 34
   related to acquired musculoskeletal disorders, 73-74
   related to congenital anomalies, 191-192

Nursing diagnoses—cont'd
    related to traumatic musculoskeletal injury, 148-149
Nursing evaluation, 43-45
Nursing process, 31-45
Nursing standards, 29
Nutrient foramen, 9

O

Oblique fracture, 151, 152
Oblique views, 62
Obturator foramen, 20
Odontoid process, 16
Older adults
    nursing care for, 30
    physical changes in, 30
Olecranon
    bursectomy of, 95-96
    cancellous bone screw in, 163
Olecranon fossa, 18
Olecranon process of ulna, 18-19
On Articulations, 3
On Fractures, 3
Open fractures, 151
Open reduction and internal fixation of metacarpal fractures,
    167-169
Operating room, patient transport to, 36
Operative arthroscopy, 75
Operative knee arthroscopy, 75-78
Orthofix external fixation device, 147
Orthofix fixator, 154
Orthopaedic implants, 57-58
Orthopaedic nurse, perioperative, role of, 5-6
Orthopaedic procedure, personnel, equipment, and supplies re-
    quired for, 36
Orthopaedic surgeon, role of, 6
Orthopaedic surgery, history of, 3-4
Orthopaedic surgical nursing, foundations of, 1-69
Orthopaedic team, 5-7
Oscillating saw blades, 56
Ossification process, 26
Osteoarthritis, arthroplasty for, 111
Osteoconductive potential, bone graft material and, 140
Osteogenic potential, bone graft material and, 140
Osteoinductive properties, bone graft material and, 140
Osteomyelitis, bacterial, 45
Osteoporosis, 27
Osteotomes, 48, 49
Osteotomy
    Chevron distal metatarsal, 135-136
    femoral
        using Coventry screw plate, 201
        using four-hole plate, 200-201
    glenoid, 103
    innominate, 202-203
    tibial, 203-207
Outcome identification, 35

P

Paré, Ambroise, 3
Passive motion devices, 67, 68, 69
Patella, 20, 21, 23
    cancellous bone screw in, 163
    circumferential wire fixation of, 161
    fracture of, repair of, 169-172
Patellar groove, 21
Patellar ligament, 23

Patellar tendon substitution, arthroscopic anterior cruciate liga-
    ment reconstruction with, 78-83
Patient
    assessment of, by perioperative nurse, 31-34
    communication with, 30-31
    implantable devices in, assessment for, 32
    medical status of, assessment of, 31
    physical condition of, assessment of, 32
    positioning of, 38-41
    postoperative complications in, 43-45
    preoperative preparation of, 32
    previous surgical procedures on, 31-32
    psychologic status of, assessment of, 32
    safety measures for, 38
    special, nursing care for, 29-30
    transport of, to operating room, 36
Patient care, planning, 35-38
Patient outcomes, identification of, 35
Patient teaching
    implementation of, 38
    planning, 35-36
Paul of Aegina, 3
Pedicles of vertebra, 15
Pelvic brim, 20
Pelvic curvature, 15
Pelvic foramina, 16
Pelvic girdle, 20-21
Pelvic inlet, 20
Pelvic outlet, 20
Pelvis, 20
Perioperative nursing, AORN quality improvement standards
    for, 43
Perioperative nursing care, 29-46
Perioperative nursing clinical practice, standards of, 29
Perioperative orthopaedic nurse, role of, 5-6
Periosteal elevators, 49
Periosteum, 9, 10
Peroneus longus muscle, 25
Personnel required for orthopaedic procedures, 36
Phalanges
    of foot, 23, 25
    of hand, 19
Phosphorus, serum, test of, 34
Physical condition of patient, assessment of, 32
Physical therapist, role of, 7
Pilot screw point, 162
Pin(s), 57, 58
    absorbable, 58
    Steinmann, for internal fixation, 161
Pin cutters, 54
Pin fixation, multiple, of femoral neck fracture, 177-178
Pin fixators, external fixation with, 154
Pisiform bone, 19
Pivot joint, 13, 14
Plan, intraoperative, 37-38
Planning in nursing process, 35-38
Plate(s), 57
    compression, fixation of forearm fracture with, 164-
        167
    compression side, and screw, insertion of, 178-182
    fixation, 146
    four-hole, femoral osteotomy using, 200-201
    for internal fixation, 163
    screw, Coventry, femoral osteotomy using, 201
Plate benders, 53
Plateau fracture, depressed, fixation of, 187-188

Pliers, 55
  bending, 53
PMMA; *see* Polymethyl methacrylate
Policies and procedures, intraoperative, 37-38
Polymethyl methacrylate, 66-67
Populations, special, nursing care for, 29-30
Portable radiographic equipment, 62
Positioning of orthopaedic patients, 38-41
Positioning devices, 64-65
Postanesthesia care unit, information given to, 69
Postoperative communication, 69
Postoperative complications, 43-45
Pott's fracture, 150
Power supplies, 65
Power-driven instruments, 55-56
Preoperative preparation of patient, 32
Preoperative procedure verification, 36
Pressure monitor, compartment, 147
Pretapped screws, 146
Previous surgical procedures, assessment of, 31-32
Procedure verification, preoperative, 36
Processes of neural arch, 15-16
Product representatives, role of, in orthopaedics, 7
Prone position, 40-41
Prostheses, 57
Prosthetic replacement
  Austin Moore, for femoral head, 173
  of shoulder for fracture, 122
Protective attire for operating room, 64
Protein, C-reactive, 34
Protractor, 55
Psychologic status of patient, assessment of, 32
Pubic symphysis, 20
Pubis, 20
Pulmonary embolism, 45
Pulsatile lavage pump, 64, 65
Pulsavac wound debridement system, 65
Pump, pulsatile lavage, 64, 65
Putti-Platt shoulder repair, 99-100

Q

Quadriceps femoris muscle, 23
Quality improvement, 43
Quality indicators, 43

R

Radial fossa, 18
Radial groove, 18
Radial tuberosity, 18
Radiographic equipment, 61-63
Radiography, 33-34
Radiologist, 7
Radiology personnel, 7
Radiology technician, 7
Radioulnar articulation, 12
Radius, 18-19
Rasps, bone, 51
Reciprocating saw blades, 56
Recon fixation device, 146
Reconstruction, anterior cruciate ligament, arthroscopic, with patellar tendon substitution, 78-83
Recumbent position, dorsal, 39
Red marrow, 9, 10
Reduction, fracture, 62
  closed, 152-153
  open, and internal fixation of metacarpal fractures, 167-169

Regional anesthesia, intravenous, 37
Regional anesthetics, 36-37
Registered nurse anesthetist, certified, 6
Registered nurse first assistant, role of, 6, 36
Release
  carpal tunnel, 94-95
    endoscopic, 86-88
  trigger finger/thumb, 92-93
Removal, disk, lumbar laminectomy for, 108-111
Repair
  of patellar fracture, 169-172
  shoulder, 97-103; *see also* Shoulder repair
  spinal, 104-111
Replacement
  hip, total, 122-129
  knee, total, 129-134
  shoulder, prosthetic, for fracture, 122
Resection, neuroma, 91-92
Resection arthroplasty, Keller, 137-138
Retracting instruments, 52, 53
Retractors, 52-53
Rheumatoid arthritis, arthroplasty for, 111
Rheumatoid factor test, 34
Rib cage, 16
Ribs, 17
Ring fixators, external fixation with, 154
RNFA; *see* Registered nurse first assistant
Rod cutters, 54
Rodding, intramedullary, of femur, 182-185
Rods, 57, 58
  for internal fixation, 163, 164
Roger Anderson pin fixator system, 154
Rongeurs, 50-51
Rotator cuff muscles, 18
Rulers, 55
Rush awl reamer, 53
Rush mallet, 54
Ruskin bone rongeur, 50
Ruskin-Liston bone-cutting forceps, 51
Russeu-Taylor interlocked fixation device, 146

S

Sacral canal, 16
Sacral crests, 16
Sacral vertebra, 14, 15, 16
Sacroiliac joint, 20
Sacrum, 16
Saddle joint, 13, 14
Safety measures for patient and personnel, 38
Sagittal saw blades, 56
Salter fracture, 151
Salter-Harris fracture, 151
Satterlee bone saw, 57
Saw(s)
  cast, 66
  manual or hand, 57
Saw blades and burs, 56
Scaphoid bone, 19
Scapula, 17-18
Schlesinger cervical rongeur, 50
Schlesinger intervertebral disk rongeur, 50
Schneider fixation device, 146
Scintigraphy, bone, 33
Scissors, wire-cutting, 54
Scoliosis, 15
"Scope of Orthopaedic Nursing Practice," 5

Screw depth gauge, 55
Screw heads, 58
Screw plate, Coventry, femoral osteotomy using, 201
Screw points, 162
Screwdrivers, 55
Screws, 57-58
  bone, 162-163
  compression side plate and, insertion of, 178-182
  for fixation, 146
  for internal fixation, 162-163
Self-tapping screws, 146, 162
Semitubular fixation plate, 146
Serum aspartate aminotransferase, 34
Serum calcium, 34
Serum phosphorus, 34
Serum uric acid, 34
Sesamoid bones, 11
Shields, leaded, for radiography, 63
Shinbone, 21
Short bones, 9, 11
Shoulder, prosthetic replacement of, for fracture, 122
Shoulder arthroscopy, 83-86
Shoulder blade, 17-18
Shoulder girdle, 17-18
Shoulder joint, 18
  arthroplasty of, 118-122
Shoulder procedures, position for, 40
Shoulder repair, 97-103
  anterior, 97-99
  Magnuson-Stack, 102
  modified Bristow-Helfet, 101
  posterior, 103
  Putti-Platt, 99-100
  Weaver-Dunn, 103
Simple subtrochanteric fracture, 175
Single-slot screw, 58
Skeletal muscle, 25
Skeletal structure, 9-25
Skeletal system, role of, 9
Skeleton
  appendicular, 11, 12
  axial, 11, 12
  structure of, 11
Skin cleansing and infection control, 42
Skull, 14
Small-bone clamp, 52
Small-fragment fixation plate, 146
Smillie retractor, 52
Smith-Petersen gouges, 49
Smooth muscle, 25
Soft tissue instruments, basic, 48
Soft tissue procedures, 91-96
Special populations, nursing care for, 29-30
Spinal anesthesia, 37
Spinal column, curves of, 15
Spinal instrumentation for congenital anomalies, 207-213
Spinal repair, 104-111
Spinous process, 15, 16
Spiral fracture, 151, 152
Splints, 67
  application of, 153
Split tibial plateau fracture, 186
Spurling rongeur, 50
Standard screw point, 162
Standards
  nursing, 29

Standards—cont'd
  of perioperative nursing clinical practice, 29
Staples, 57, 58
Steinmann pins for internal fixation, 161
Sternum, 16, 17
Stille-Horsley bone-cutting forceps, 51
Stille-Liston bone-cutting forceps, 51
Stille-Luer bone rongeur, 50
Stimulation
  bone, 142
  bone graft and, 140-142
Stimulator
  fusion site, insertion of, 142
  long-bone, insertion of, 142
Styloid process of ulna, 18, 19
Subarachnoid block, 37
Subscapular muscle, 18
Substitution, patellar tendon, arthroscopic anterior cruciate ligament reconstruction with, 78-83
Subtrochanteric fractures, 172, 175, 176
Suction systems, 64
Superior articular process, 15, 16
Supine position, 39, 40
Supplies
  equipment and, 61-69
  required for orthopaedic procedures, 36
Support personnel, assistive, role of, 7
Supraglenoid tubercle, 17
Supraspinous muscle, 18
Surgeon, orthopaedic, role of, 6
Surgery
  orthopaedic, history of, 3-4
  previous, assessment of, 31-32
Surgical interventions, 71-213
Surgical neck of humerus, 18
Surgical nursing, orthopaedic, foundations of, 1-69
Surgical technologist, certified, role of, 6
Suture joints, 12
Swan neck gouge, 49
Swayback; *see* Lordosis
Symphysis, 12
  pubic, 20
Synarthroses, 11, 12
Synarthrotic joints, 11, 12
Synchondrosis, 12
Syndesmoses, 12
Synovial fluid, 12
Synovial membrane, 13
Synovium, 12

T

Table, fracture, 65, 147
Talipes equinovarus, 193
  correction of, 193, 194-197
Talus bone, 23, 25
Tarsal bones, 23, 25
Taylor spinal retractor, 53
Teaching, patient
  implementation of, 38
  planning, 35-36
Team
  anesthesia, role of, 6
  orthopaedic, 5-7
Teardrop fracture, 151
Technician, radiology, 7
Technologist, surgical, certified, role of, 6

Tendon(s), 9
   patellar, substitution of, arthroscopic anterior cruciate ligament
      reconstruction with, 78-83
Teres minor muscle, 18
Tests
   blood, 33
   required before orthopaedic procedures, 32-34
Therapist, physical, role of, 7
Thoracic curvature, 15
Thoracic vertebrae, 14, 15, 16
Thoracic vertebral bodies, 16
Thorax, 16-17
Three-point positioner, 65
Thromboembolic disease, 44-45
Thromboembolism, 44-45
Thrombosis, venous, deep, 44-45
Thumb, 19
   trigger, release of, 92-93
Tibia, 20, 21-22, 23
   bone graft of, 142
   cancellous bone screw in, 163
Tibial osteotomy, 203-207
Tibial plateau fractures, management of, 186
Tibial tuberosity, 21, 22, 23
Tibiofibular articulation, 12
Tissue structure, 9
TOD fixation plate, 146
Tomography, computed, 33
Total elbow joint arthroplasty, 113-118
Total hip replacement, 122-129
Total knee replacement, 129-134
Tourniquets, 63-64
   application of, 63
   cuff lengths for, 63
   duration of use of, 64
Townley femur caliper, 55
Trabeculae, 9
Transport, patient, to operating room, 36
Transverse arch of foot, 23, 25
Transverse fracture, 151, 152
Transverse process, 15
Trapezium bone, 19
Trapezoid bone, 19
Traumatic musculoskeletal injury, 145-189
   instruments to treat, 145-147
   nursing care for, 145
   nursing diagnoses related to, 148-149
Trigger finger/thumb release, 92-93
Triquetrum bone, 19
Trocar screw point, 162
Trochanters, 21
Trochlea of humerus, 18
Trochlear notch, 19
Trochoid joint, 13, 14
True pelvis, 20
True ribs, 17
Trunk, muscles of, 24
Tubercle, greater and lesser, 18
Tuberosity
   iliac, 20

Tuberosity—cont'd
   radial, 18
   tibial, 21, 22, 23

U
Ulna, 18-19
Ulnar notch, 18
Unifix external fixation device, 147
Upper extremity, 18-19
   muscles of, 25
Uric acid, serum, 34

V
Vacpac, 65
Vacuum pack, 65
Venography, 34
Venous thrombosis, deep, 44-45
Verbrugge bone-holding forceps, 51
Vertebrae, 14, 15
   structure of, 15
   types of, 14
Vertebral bodies, thoracic, 16
Vertebral canal, 15
Vertebral column, 14-16
Vertebral deviation, treatment of
   using Cotrell Doubesset technique, 207-211
   using Luque technique, 211-213
Vertebral foramen, 15
Video systems, 64
Volkmann's canals, 9, 10

W
Wagner pin fixator system, 154
Weaver-Dunn shoulder repair, 103
Weitlaner retractor, 53
Williams fixation device, 146
Wire cutters, 54
Wire fixation, circumferential, 161
Wire-cutting scissors, 54
Wires, 57, 58
   Kirschner, 58
Woodruff head screw, 58
Wormian bones, 11
Wound debridement system, 65
Wound drainage systems, 67
Wound infections, 45
Wrist, 19

X
Xenografts, 140
Xeroform, 67
Xiphoid process, 17

Y
Yellow marrow, 9, 10
Y-nail, 146

Z
Zielke modification of Dwyer instrumentation, 213
Zielke procedure, 213